When Down Syndrome and Autism Intersect

When Down Syndrome and Autism Intersect

A Guide to DS-ASD for Parents and Professionals

Margaret Froehlke, R.N. & Robin Zaborek

Woodbine House   2013

Comsewogue Public Library
170 Terryville Road
Port Jefferson Station, NY 11776

© 2013 Margaret Froehlke and Robin Zaborek

First edition

All rights reserved. Published in the United States of America by Woodbine House,
6510 Bells Mill Road, Bethesda, MD 20817. 800-843-7323. www.woodbinehouse.com

Library of Congress Cataloging in Publication Data

Froehlke, Margaret.
 When Down syndrome and autism intersect : a guide to DS-ASD for parents and professionals / edited
by Margaret Froehlke & Robin Zaborek. — First edition.
  pages cm
 Includes bibliographical references and index.
 ISBN 978-1-60613-160-2
 1. Children with mental disabilities—Care. 2. Developmentally disabled children—Care 3. Autism in
children. 4. Down syndrome. I. Zaborek, Robin. II. Title.
 RJ506.M4F69 2012
 362.4—dc23
         2012031669

Manufactured in the United States of America

10 9 8 7 6 5 4 3 2 1

This book is dedicated to the loving memories of
Janet Kay Zaborek and Dr. Elina Manghi

Table of Contents

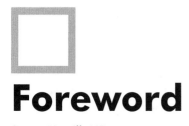

Foreword

Susan Merrill, MD

When Robin Zaborek gave birth to her second son, I was her pediatrician and was asked by the nursery pediatrician if I would give Robin the difficult news that Tommy was born with Down syndrome. Even though I was nervous, I already had an established relationship with Robin and felt it would be best if the news came from me. I had been a pediatrician for three years, and this was my first experience working with a family with a child with Down syndrome.

When I delivered the news, Robin said, "I can handle it but I'm not sure my husband can." Yet when I talked to her husband, Bob, he said he could handle it but he wasn't sure about Robin. When they both said the same thing about their spouses, I knew they were going to be fine.

Several years later, Robin and Bob considered adopting a baby, Janet Kay, who also had Down syndrome. Besides having other problems, including being born without a left hand and with an imperforate anus, Janet Kay had severe pulmonary hypertension, with the potential for significant heart disease that could cause her to die prematurely. In an honest discussion with Robin about the cardiologist's pessimistic report, as well as Janet Kay's other problems, I asked Robin if she understood the magnitude of Janet Kay's medical problems. But by that time, she and Bob had fallen in love with this baby. And so, between Tommy and Janet Kay, Robin became my teacher about children with chronic special needs.

It is hard for a doctor to admit she doesn't know everything about her patients' diagnoses. That's why it's so important for healthcare professionals to listen to what parents tell you about their children—who they are with 24 hours a day. After Tommy was born, Robin taught herself about Down syndrome, enough so that when Janet Kay started exhibiting symptoms not associated with Down syndrome, such as flapping her arms and not making eye contact, she wondered if her daughter had autism. Robin had to bring her concerns up with me at several office visits before I referred her to a specialist. In hindsight, I wish we had recognized the autism earlier, but in one office visit, many other concerns are raised and there's a limited amount of time.

After the initial evaluation, the specialist determined that Janet Kay, then age 4, didn't have autism. But Robin continued to be struck by how different Janet Kay was from other children with Down syndrome. She came back to me when Janet Kay was 10, and said, "I think she needs to be reevaluated." It was then that we learned that Janet Kay indeed had a co-occurrence of Down syndrome and autism spectrum disorder (DS-ASD).

As discussed in Chapter One, it's only in the past 10 to 20 years that we've learned that up to 18 percent of persons with Down syndrome will also have autism or ASD. This is information that most healthcare professionals are not aware of and underscores the importance of this reference guide. The earlier that ASD is discovered in a child with Down syndrome, the sooner critical interventions can begin. Now, starting at 18 months, pediatricians screen every child for autism. Doctors are starting to realize that with dual diagnoses, the medical issues become more complicated. For example, kids with Down syndrome have an increased risk of celiac disease. The pediatrician needs to be mindful of these connections.

Although the progress that is being made in terms of our awareness about these disabilities is important, what I learned from Robin is the importance of a partnership between the health professional and the parents. As a doctor, you often focus on one problem at a time, so it's sometimes hard to see the bigger picture. It's especially hard with kids who have multiple problems, like DS-ASD, which is why parent input can be so helpful. Parents are the ones who see their children's behavior day in and day out.

At the same time, health professionals can't keep up with all the evolving medical knowledge. That's where parents like Robin Zaborek and Margaret Froehlke come in. In their quests to do as much as possible for their children, they learn everything they can, and, in the process, become advocates. Robin and Margaret started a support group for other parents who are dealing with DS-ASD, and the two of them (along with Sarah Hartway) have put together an annual conference via the Down Syndrome-Autism Connection™, bringing together parents and specialists. All we doctors need to do is listen to these parents.

It's a lot easier to collaborate with parents if you have the kind of relationship I have with Robin. I trusted her enough to show my ignorance about the subject of DS-ASD. One of the most satisfying things about being a pediatrician is developing an honest relationship with parents, so you can say, "I don't really have the expertise with that, but I know people who do, and I can refer you." This is also where the concept of medical home (discussed in Chapter Six) is so important, because a team consisting of the doctor, chronic special needs nurses, and others can form a partnership in assessing and working with those with special needs.

As caretaker and doctor, Robin and I have journeyed together for over 26 years. I applaud her—and Margaret—on the next step of this journey. Because their knowledge comes from experience as well as from educating themselves, their book is a great resource for both health professionals and families, especially for those parents who don't know where to turn.

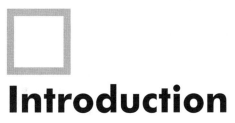

Introduction

Margaret Froehlke and Robin Zaborek

As parents of teens with co-occurring Down syndrome and autism spectrum disorders (DS-ASD), we conceived this book because there was little available to guide us during the time when our children were first exhibiting autism behaviors, during the diagnosis phase, and beyond. We remember the heartache and isolation of not quite fitting in with the greater Down syndrome community. We remember wondering why our children were not developing like their peers with Down syndrome, even though we felt like we were working twice as hard as other parents with fewer results. We dreamed of a resource guide to help families and professionals alike, so that their journeys would not be as scary, frustrating, and difficult as ours were.

When Down Syndrome and Autism Intersect: A Guide to DS-ASD for Parents and Professionals was written collaboratively by specialists who may be parents and/or experts in their field on Down syndrome, autism, and/or the combination of the two. The topics discussed cover the lifespan and provide valuable information and data that is current, evidenced-based, and valuable for improving the lives of people with DS-ASD, as well as helpful to those who love and care for them.

For many of you, this topic may be a brand new concept. Parents who are reading this book may have just received the diagnosis of autism in their child with Down syndrome and want to learn as much as possible about how autism may affect their loved one. Many parents report that even though they have suspected autism for a while, upon diagnosis they feel as if their world has been turned upside down *again*, and they may grieve intensely. Others may be in disbelief that their child could possibly receive a second major diagnosis and wonder about the odds of this happening to them. And still other parents, who are dealing with multiple medical conditions on top of the Down syndrome and autism, may feel like, "Why not? He has everything else!"

Healthcare providers, school personnel, and others who may be new to DS-ASD might be at a loss about how to help the families in their care. We sincerely hope that this book will be a valuable resource to you in your workplace.

We believe that it is imperative to spread awareness of co-occurring Down syndrome and autism spectrum disorders. We also believe that it is vital to increase compassion and understanding for individuals with DS-ASD, their families, and the professionals who serve them, with the ultimate goal of enabling our loved ones to live healthy, safe, and joyful lives. It is our desire that every single family member and professional caring for a child or adult with DS-ASD will get the support they need and come to the clear realization that they are not alone.

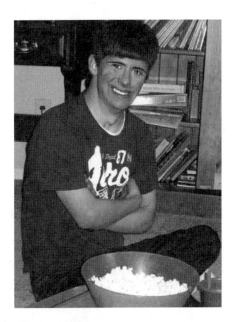

1

Introduction to the DS-ASD Diagnosis
One Family's Journey

Robert Froehlke, MD, and Margaret Froehlke, RN, BSN

Not that many years ago, it was thought that people with Down syndrome only rarely, if ever, also had autism. In fact, some suggested that individuals with Down syndrome were somehow "protected" from developing autism (Turk, 1992). In the past 10 to 20 years, however, more studies have been done showing that anywhere from 5 to 39 percent of individuals with Down syndrome (DS) will also have autism or Autism Spectrum Disorder (ASD) (Moss, 2009; DiGuiseppi, 2010). This wide range of incidences reflects not only the variability of diagnostic criteria used for ASD in these studies, but also the wide overlap of the core symptoms of ASD with those of cognitive impairment and intellectual disability well characterized in Down syndrome (Molloy, 2009; DiGuiseppi, 2010; Gray, 2011; Lowenthal, 2010; Ji, 2011). Practically, this means that the recognition and diagnosis of ASD in Down syndrome is typically delayed, and that autistic symptoms are often attributed to the child's intellectual impairment, rather than to a diagnosis of both DS and ASD.

Making a diagnosis of autism in a child with Down syndrome is important for several reasons. First, though some of the developmental issues with autism and DS are similar (such as speech delay and being more visual learners), other areas of development and behavior are very different. One of the areas of strength in many people with Down syndrome is their social interactiveness (Cooper, 2009). This is in contrast to the person with DS-ASD, whose social interactions are impaired (see Chapter 3). Second, the approach to educating children with both DS and ASD will often be different than it is for children who have just DS and cognitive impairment. Children with DS-ASD not only need to have their academics attended to, but also their social skills. It is for this reason that inclusion with typical peers in the school is very important. (See Chapter 12 on education.) Finally, behavior problems are very common in children and adults with DS-ASD, which is often the reason the diagnosis is made (Lott, 2010; Esbensen, 2010). Methods used in addressing behavior problems in children and adults with autism, such as Applied Behavior Analysis (ABA) (see Chapter 11), should also be used in the child with DS-ASD.

Physical and medical issues generally are going to be similar for the person with both DS and ASD and the person with just DS, but mental health and behavioral issues are often going to be more similar to those of a person with ASD. Thus it is important that all those involved in the life of a person with DS-ASD—parents, teachers, caretakers, medical providers, and other professionals—keep both perspectives in mind. The story of our son Brennan, and our journey with him, is illustrative of these issues. Brennan is 17 years old and has Down syndrome-Autism Spectrum Disorder (DS-ASD).

Brennan is the third of our four children. He has older siblings, Elizabeth and Alex, and a younger sister, Sarah. Brennan was diagnosed with Down syndrome (DS) at birth. Brennan was the first member of any of our immediate or extended families to have Down syndrome. Considering that Robert is one of 5 children, Margaret is one of 12 children and has over 70 first cousins, and Brennan has over 30 first cousins, it is actually somewhat surprising that he was the first person with Down syndrome in our combined families. Prior to Brennan's birth, our experience with persons with Down syndrome was minimal, even though both of us are healthcare providers. Needless to say, we immediately began learning everything we could to better understand Down syndrome. We devoured books and articles, joined support groups, and learned about educational programs that had anything to do with supporting persons with Down syndrome.

Becoming well informed proved to be the best way to be an advocate for Brennan, even among our own families and friends. As most new parents of a child with special needs do, we too found it emotionally exhausting to care for our new child with special needs, and become "experts" in the diagnosis, along with caring for the rest of our children.   Thankfully, as a baby, Brennan was physically very healthy. Newborns with DS are at risk for several serious health issues, including congenital heart disease, gastrointestinal (GI) malformations, and feeding and growth problems. Brennan did have a minor heart defect (a small atrial septal defect) which closed by itself within his first year of life. His GI system was normal, but he did have significant feeding difficulties. For the first three months of his life, Margaret both nursed Brennan and pumped breast milk every two hours. Added to this sleepless routine were special oral nursing aides to encourage Brennan to suck. Worrying about Brennan's weight gain and his ability to nurse was our main concern those first three months. Once we successfully got over the nursing hurdle, we began focusing all of our attention on Brennan's developmental milestones and his personalized therapy program.

A great resource for children with developmental delays is a federally mandated program for early intervention services, beginning at birth. We then lived in Michigan and Brennan was enrolled in Michigan's early intervention services program, Early On. Through Early On, children receive state-funded therapy services as early as six weeks of age. Brennan had a therapy coordinator, a physical therapist, an occupational therapist, and a speech and language therapist. The team of therapists visited us two days a week, rotating therapy services. We also attended a monthly playgroup through Early On. Families who were in the Early On program met with their children for a therapist-facilitated playgroup/therapy session. This monthly meeting provided a wonderful opportunity to get to meet other families with children with developmental disabilities, as well as to observe how other children with DS were progressing.

Our lives were very busy managing Brennan's therapy schedule and staying on top of our other two children's schedules. We carefully tracked Brennan's progress. By early November 1993, Brennan was able to hold his head up and roll over, and he was cooing and vocalizing all the time. He was showing great progress in his attempts at sitting up. His overall development was still within the range of a typical child's milestones. That was until late November, 1993, when Brennan was just 5 months old.

Unexpected Concerns

It was just after Thanksgiving when Margaret began to notice Brennan was frequently doing what she thought was the "Moro" reflex (startling). She mentioned this observation to her husband, Bob (he is a pediatrician). He was concerned because infants should have outgrown the Moro reflex by this age. The next day, Bob was home when this unusual movement of Brennan's occurred. Bob was immediately alarmed and told Margaret that he thought Brennan was having a type of seizures called Infantile Spasms. This particular seizure disorder is typically extremely difficult to control, and usually causes the child to have long-lasting devastating neurologic outcomes, and sometimes even death.

We went through a traumatic few weeks of CT scans, PET Scans, EEGs, and administering injections of a medicine called ACTH into our little baby Brennan. It seemed as if the treatment and the seizures would kill him. Neither of the specialists who treated Brennan offered us much hope. Fortunately, after much concentrated prayer and faith, Brennan's health improved. Our faith kept us strong and hopeful.

Once Brennan's seizure activity stopped, we began to notice that he had completely lost many of his prior developmental gains. We started over with all his therapy goals and watched him slowly make progress. Following this post-seizure time, Brennan's development began to include atypical behavior that was different from the typical behavior of his same-aged peers with DS. Our therapy team also observed Brennan's behavior and agreed that it was peculiar or strange as compared to other children with DS with whom they were working. One atypical behavior that we noticed was Brennan's complete fixation on making shadows with his hands by holding them out over the floor using the light in the room to make shadows. He also was fascinated watching any and all ceiling fans. Breaking his attention from either of these activities was impossible; we learned to work around them.

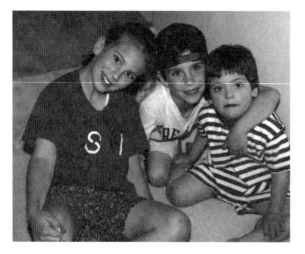

Prior to the Infantile Spasms, Brennan had constantly made cooing and vocalizing noises. However, in the post-seizure time, he remained silent. It was also harder to engage him with eye contact, or to attract his attention using our voices, although hearing tests were within normal limits. We found the best way to get his attention and to settle him down was through quietly singing familiar calming songs to him. At that time, we felt these changes and losses in his development were temporary, and due to the intensity of his seizures and medical treatment. We did not realize then that the behaviors we were observing not only were permanent, but were harbingers of autism. It is now known that seizures in persons with Down syndrome can be associated with cognitive decline and autism (Lott, 2010; Molloy, Murray, 2009).

As Brennan approached his first birthday, we noticed that certain voices and sounds really upset him. Bob's voice and laughter were among the most stressful. When Bob would laugh, or even speak, Brennan would often go into a meltdown of screaming. Nothing would settle him down except Bob's silence. We searched for answers to help us with these unsettling behaviors through our network of parents we knew who had children with DS, our therapy team, Down syndrome literature, and through our pediatrician and school professionals. When Brennan was three years old, we asked our pediatrician for his help with strategies to help stop the screaming. He suggested we tape record Brennan's screaming and play it back to him. He also recommended that we use a blow-horn whenever Brennan screamed. We took these recommendations in stride and actually tried them, with mixed results.

Brennan was slower to walk than the typical child with DS. He walked independently at 30 months. Once he was mobile, however, it wasn't long before he used this new skill to run away from us at will. Because he was so quiet, we wouldn't immediately realize he was gone until it was too late. There were several frightening experiences where we found him around the block from our home, wandering. As time went on, we noticed he tended to escape more often when we were having conversations with other adults. To this day, conversations between adults are still hard for him, and are a trigger for him to bolt. We think that conversations increase his anxiety because of their unpredictable nature in length and voice fluctuations, including laughter and raised voices.

Once Brennan entered into our public school preschool program, he began having aggressive behavior problems, including biting and hitting his classmates. While we were at an IEP meeting discussing how to address this challenging behavior, the school principal actually recommended we get some "cat toys" for Brennan, and that we put him in a "pen." This suggestion greatly offended us and made it even harder to feel we were on the right path to solving these issues.

These examples are offered not to criticize the professionals' poor advice, but to show that with all the best intentions, our search to find answers was unsuccessful—even with other professionals who knew Brennan. Our own feelings of isolation and worry grew.

For several more years, Brennan continued on in school, struggling with transitions, behaviors, sensory issues, communication, and social interactions. He was extremely sensitive to any and all changes. Wearing new footgear would lead to a "sit-in" for two days; getting a haircut, going to the dentist, and having blood drawn were sources of extreme anxiety; crowds, game buzzers, bells, alarms, sleeping away from home on family trips, and seeing/hearing someone crying, to name a few, were constant sources of stress for Brennan—and, in turn, for all of us—and would often lead to meltdowns for Brennan.

For much of the time, we were unable to detect which triggers upset him and/or caused meltdowns. We lived through many horrible public scenes of aggression, screaming, and running away. Going anywhere with Brennan was both unpredictable and extremely stressful for our whole family. Holidays, family gatherings, and get-togethers with friends are usually events that families look forward to and enjoy. For us, these occasions were sources of stress, worry, and anxiety. As a consequence, we often declined invitations from others, and our family became more socially isolated.

As our everyday life with Brennan was full of meltdowns and behavior outbursts, the nights offered no reprieve. We were exhausted from the 'round-the-clock attention Brennan demanded. For the first six years of his life, he did not sleep through the night. We tried everything from regular daytime naps and bedtime routines to getting custom-made blackout shades in his bedroom. Nothing seemed to work. Starting before midnight, Brennan would begin running in circles in his room. When we would come in to help him get back in bed, he would get upset because he wanted to run. We were on the verge of despair when we learned that some children with autism who had sleep problems improved with a supplement—melatonin. We decided to try it, and within a few days Brennan slept through the night for the first time in six years!

Getting the Autism Diagnosis

It was increasingly clear that what Brennan had was more than just Down syndrome; we began to think that he also had autism. An article by Joan Medlen (*Disability Solutions,* Volume 3, Issues 5 & 6) was extremely helpful for us. The article shared the story of Joan's teenaged son who had DS-ASD. It was the first piece of literature that rang true about Brennan. It provided a bright ray of hope for us! We shared the article with Brennan's IEP team and pediatrician, and the strategies and recommendations in the article were incorporated into Brennan's IEP. These interventions had an immediate, quick, and positive impact. We then proceeded to have Brennan formally evaluated to see if he was indeed autistic. We did this not only to confirm our suspicions, but also because our school district required students to have a formal diagnosis of autism in order to receive services from the district's Autism Consultant. A complete evaluation done in the fall of 1999 by the regional expert in autism, diagnosed Brennan with Pervasive Developmental Disorder Not Otherwise Specified (PDD NOS); this is now referred to as Autism Spectrum Disorder (ASD).

For many families, it would have been a blow to learn that their child had ASD, but for us, it was actually a relief. We finally had an explanation as to why Brennan was different from other children with Down syndrome. It not only gave us an explanation for his atypical behaviors, but also gave us direction on how to address his most difficult and disruptive behaviors. We learned that the teaching methods and strategies used with ASD were very different from those used with children with just DS. This gave us hope that things would improve for Brennan.

Officially knowing that Brennan had both Down syndrome and autism did help; however, it didn't suddenly "fix" him. For many years, Brennan's life outside of the school day was still very volatile. It was hard for us to read his cues or triggers, and we didn't have a dedicated family member constantly available to monitor him and assess his environment/reactions.

At first, we chose to handle challenging social or public settings by avoiding them. One of us would routinely stay home with Brennan while the rest of the family went on with the typical activities of family life. We thought this arrangement would be the only way to avoid having to deal with the aftermath of meltdowns and would best serve Brennan. Our "avoidance strategy" worked in the short-run to keep Brennan on an even keel; however, it also led to feelings of further isolation and sorrow for both Brennan and our whole family. Brennan became our "hidden child." Many of our friends and community members didn't know we had a fourth child. And, Brennan was not gaining any skills to handle social situations outside of our immediate family, home, or school. We realized we had to rethink this strategy to make things better in the long run, and to help Brennan adapt to the real world.

Strategies for Success

Thankfully, we gained incredible support from Brennan's IEP team and school specialists, who offered ideas and strategies to take small steps toward acclimating Brennan to the world outside our doors. We also met with a psychologist familiar with behavior problems in children with autism and other developmental disabilities. He helped us to form a behavior plan for Brennan, based upon Applied Behavior Analysis (ABA) principles. The behavior plan proved to not only be a useful tool for us to follow at home, but also at school, where it was incorporated into his IEP. It formed the foundation and cornerstone for how his future teachers and para-professionals assisted him and helped prevent and ameliorate difficult behaviors.

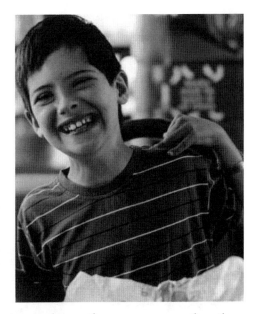

Over many months and years, Brennan made slow progress in his ability to handle social situations. It took many years to heighten our own level of sensitivity so that we could perceive what things heightened Brennan's anxiety and how to successfully prepare for and react to them. As these triggers became more obvious to us, we began to achieve success in creating environments for Brennan that worked. As our ability to provide successful strategies grew, so did Brennan's ability to handle new situations. Strategies such as adequate preparation time for transitions, offering visual and auditory cues before transitions, singing familiar songs to decrease anxiety in difficult situations, and selecting settings that held fewer potential triggers were all part of our autism behavior arsenal.

Brennan's inclusion with typical peers also proved to be very helpful. Brennan identified more and more with his peers and wanted to be with them. Though he was clearly different than his typical peers in school, they began to include Brennan as a fellow classmate. These methods led to more predictable success in Brennan's ability to handle different and strange situations. With these new successes, we began exposing Brennan to more and varied settings. Over time and with some setbacks, Brennan began to participate in increasingly more difficult and complex social situations. Though we have had, and continue to have, some failures and meltdowns in social situations, using this approach we have also had some notable successes, a few of which we share below.

When Brennan was 11 years old, his younger sister, Sarah, was preparing for her First Communion. Attending church had been one of the most difficult social situations for Brennan, and we had not really thought about Brennan receiving his First Communion in the traditional way—with a large group ceremony. When Margaret saw Brennan praying in his room, however, she felt he might be ready, and had him join Sarah in some of her class's preparations. He met her class and practiced with them—processing into church and tasting unconsecrated hosts. He did well in these activities, so we decided to have him try to take his First Communion with Sarah.

On the actual First Communion Day, the church was packed with First Communicants, families, and visitors. Normally, this setting would have been an obvious one to avoid for Brennan. However, we held our breath and counted on Brennan's keen interest in following and imitating his peers. Brennan lined up as he had done in practice with Sarah's class. He was the very last in line, with Sarah as his partner, and made his way slowly, reverently up the aisle. He was a little behind the rest of the group, but having been conveniently paired with Sarah, he would look at her for reassurance, and he successfully made his way up to meet the priest and received Communion for the first time! Although our nerves were still on edge, we felt a great sense of joy and accomplishment at how well he had done on this BIG day! From that day forward, Brennan has received Communion each weekend.

A similar strategy was used in teaching Brennan to participate with typical peers in sports. Though Brennan has been, and continues to be, an active participant in Special Olympics, we also wanted him to participate in sports with typical peers. Brennan liked running, and when he was in the sixth grade, he joined the school cross country team. The coach and school supported his participation and provided a high

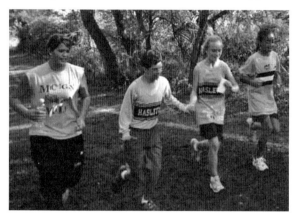

school volunteer to support Brennan. Brennan practiced weekly with his school's cross-country team. His teammates were very attentive to him. They would include him in parts of their run, and remember to take time to use encouraging words and high fives to keep him moving.

When the time came for Brennan's first cross country meet, we were all very anxious. Now, along with his familiar teammates, there were over 100 other noisy participants and their fans gathered. Again, this would normally have been a situation that Brennan would have run away FROM, rather than run WITH. However, with the gentle support of the high school volunteer, and the encouragement of his teammates, Brennan lined up for the start. The gun went off, and so did the 100-plus runners, with Brennan among them!

We followed the spectators and families to the finish line, and anxiously waited for Brennan. Soon the fastest runners appeared, running out from the wooded trail; then more and more runners crossed the finish line—Brennan nowhere in sight. Finally, Bob discreetly went looking for him and found him on the trail with his volunteer about 400 yards short of the finish line. Just as Bob was about to intercede, he heard a lot of voices coming from the trail ahead . . . . It was a group of his teammates coming to get Brennan to bring him to the finish line! They called to him and encouraged him to join them. Suddenly Brennan was in the center of about a dozen classmates, running with them toward the finish line. He was the last runner across the tape, but the audience's cheers for him were the loudest. The fans in the stands, regardless of which school, were cheering him on! Tears were streaming down the faces of people who didn't even know who he was. It was a Hallmark Movie moment. Brennan was beaming!

It occurred to us that one of the most powerful tools that helped Brennan push himself through new and challenging social situations was feeling included by his peers. Brennan was not so different from other kids in this regard. The power of peers was unmistakable. If he was aligned with a peer to do anything, amazing things could happen. We have continued to optimize the use of peers as often as possible. Brennan now participates as an altar server at our church through a peer-supported program. Being creative by using a combination of successful strategies and methods has allowed Brennan the opportunities to be successful in many different situations. He participates in special physical education programs at his school, general education sports activities, and Special Olympic activities. He runs track with his regular high school track team; has learned to ski with an adapted ski program; plays basketball with his high school's Special Olympics team; swims on his neighborhood swim team, and enjoys going to school dances. We would never have dreamed or hoped so much could have changed for the better with Brennan over such a relatively short time.

At the writing of this chapter, Brennan is on the threshold of entering adulthood. Brennan and our family have come a long way in learning to live with both his diagnoses of Down syndrome and autism.

Though Brennan's story is obviously unique to him and our family, many aspects of his life and our journey with him are demonstrative of important features in persons with DS-ASD; not only regarding some of the challenges the diagnosis brings, but also some of the successes in approaching those challenges. First, our son had the seizure disorder of Infantile Spasms. Seizures now are recognized as being more common in persons with Down syndrome who also have autism, and thus when someone with Down syndrome develops seizures, it is important not only to treat the seizure disorder, but to be on the watch for characteristics that suggest autism. Second, our son had regression of developmental milestones, following his seizures. This is commonly seen in children with autism (Castillo, 2008), and thus should raise it as a possible diagnosis. Third, as described above, Brennan developed many behaviors that are more often seen in persons with autism:

    a. stereotypes of fixation with shadows or dangling objects;
    b. sensory processing problems, such as his responses to loud noises, medical exams/testing, trying new footgear, or having his hair cut;
    c. elopement and running away;
    d. sleep difficulties;
    e. social aversiveness and difficulties in crowds;
    f. meltdowns and severe tantrums at changes or disruptions in routines.

Though many of these behaviors may be seen in people with developmental delays, when they do exist, one needs to again consider the possibility of a diagnosis of ASD.

Finally, getting to the diagnosis took several years in our son. The diagnosis of ASD is not rare in persons with Down syndrome, affecting at least 5 percent or more. Thus, it is important to consider the diagnosis when a person with Down syndrome has the characteristics above. More recent studies have shown that the use of diagnostic tools can distinguish children with Down syndrome and autism from those who are not autistic (Ji, 2011). Making the diagnosis is important. We found that, although it was not easy news to receive that our son had ASD, it at least gave us direction and an

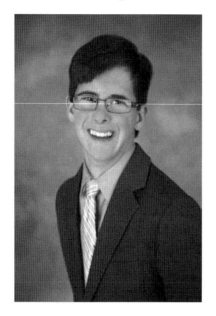

approach to his education and treating his behaviors. As our story illustrates, our son's successes in overcoming or ameliorating many of his challenges have, in large part, been due to using educational and behavioral strategies used for autism; strategies such as applied behavior analysis, visual prompts, awareness of anxiety triggers, and peer support.

Our journey has been a roller coaster at times, without a guide map or directions. At times we stumbled along with only our undying love for Brennan keeping us strong. In the early days, we often felt depressed and hopeless, but thankfully we made it through those tumultuous years, and now have days that are fairly predictable and peaceful. As with all individuals with DS-ASD, Brennan has a unique set of triggers that needed to be identified and supported for him to become successful in any given situation.

For us, the combination of providing the supports Brennan needs to deal with his autism, and then capitalizing on his nature with DS to be a social person, has given him opportunities to be known in his community and to feel a sense of accomplishment and pride in many areas. As a family, the joy and pride we each feel when Brennan overcomes these challenges is immeasurable. Though having a child with co-occurring Down syndrome and autism is difficult and challenging, there are also many joys—particularly the joy in knowing that Brennan has positively impacted the community at large in their feelings of respect and dignity for people of all abilities.

References

Castillo, H., Patterson, B., Hickey, F., Kinsman, A., Howard, J.M., Mitchell, T., & Molloy, C.A. (2008). Difference in age at regression in children with autism with and without Down syndrome. *Journal of Developmental and Behavioral Pediatrics 29(2):* 89-93.

Cooper, S.A. & van der Speck, R. (2009). Epidemiology of mental ill health in adults with intellectual disabilities. *Current Opinion in Psychiatry 22(5):* 431-6.

DiGuiseppi, C., Hepburn, S., Davis, J.M., Fidler, D.J., Hartway, S., Lee, N.R., Miller, L., Ruttenber, M., & Robinson, C. (2010). Screening for autism spectrum disorders in children with Down syndrome: Population prevalence and screening test characteristics. *Journal of Developmental and Behavioral Pediatrics 31(3):* 181-91.

Esbensen, A.J., Bishop, S., Seltzer, M.M., Greenberg, J.S., & Taylor, J.L. (2010). Comparisons between individuals with autism spectrum disorders and individuals with Down syndrome in adulthood. *American Journal on Intellectual and Developmental Disabilities 115(4):* 277-90.

Gray, L., Ansell, P., Baird, G., & Parr, J.R. (2011). The continuing challenge of diagnosing autism spectrum disorder in children with Down syndrome. *Child: Care, Health, and Development 37(4):* 459-61.

Ji, N.Y., Capone, G.T., & Kaufmann, W.E. (2011). Autism spectrum disorder in Down syndrome: Cluster analysis of Aberrant Behaviour Checklist data supports diagnosis. *Journal of Intellectual Disability Research 55 (11):* 1064–77.

Lott, I.T. & Dierssen, M. (2010). Cognitive deficits and associated neurological complications in individuals with Down's syndrome. *The Lancet Neurology 9(6):* 623-33.

Lowenthal, R., Mercadante, M.T., Belisário Filho, J.F., Pilotto, R.F., & de Paula, CS. (2010). Autism spectrum disorder in Down syndrome: Definition of the cutoff point for the autism screening questionnaire screening instrument. *Journal of Developmental and Behavioral Pediatrics 31(8):* 684.

Molloy, C.A., Murray, D.S., Kinsman, A., Castillo, H., Mitchell, T., Hickey, F.J., & Patterson, B. (2009). Differences in the clinical presentation of Trisomy 21 with and without autism. *Journal of Intellectual Disability Research 53(2):* 143-51.

Moss, J. & Howlin, P. (2009). Autism spectrum disorders in genetic syndromes: Implications for diagnosis, intervention and understanding the wider autism spectrum disorder population. *Journal of Intellectual Disability Research 53(10):* 852-73.

Turk, J. (1992). The fragile X syndrome: On the way to a behavioural phenotype. *British Journal of Psychiatry 160:* 24–35.

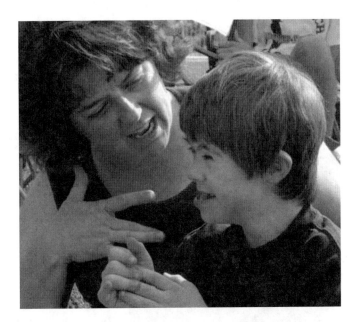

2

But I Was Just Getting Used to Holland
Adjusting to the Autism Diagnosis

Sarah A. Hartway, RN, MS

Virtually every parent of a child with Down syndrome remembers when they first heard that diagnosis. For most, this was a life-changing moment. Some learned months prior to birth, some learned shortly before birth, and most learned soon after their child's birth. While the reaction and emotions in that moment vary, almost all parents experienced some degree of confusion and fear. For some there was joy; for many there was shock and sadness.

The adjustment parents experience when learning that their child has Down syndrome can be complex and lengthy. This is a topic that has been researched and reported, so we know some things about parental grief and adaptation. We also know that the majority of these parents come to a point of adaptation that allows them to see the wonder that is their child and to experience the special joy that comes in raising a child with Down syndrome.

Most new or expectant parents whose child has Down syndrome come across the 1987 essay by Emily Perl Kingsley, "Welcome to Holland." In the essay a metaphor is employed to demonstrate the differences a parent experiences in raising a child with Down syndrome as compared to the child they may have pictured raising. The metaphor describes a traveler expecting to visit Italy, but finding herself in Holland instead.

Initially there is confusion and sadness, but eventually the pleasures of the unexpected destination are appreciated. For some new parents of children with Down syndrome, this metaphor is an apt description of their experiences.

In the early days, weeks, and months, comfort and hope can come in a number of forms. Some are comforted by the words of others. Many find comfort in the support of 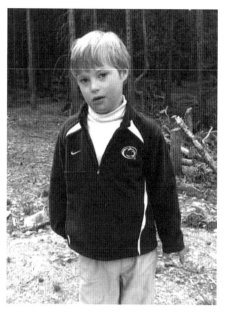 other parents of children with Down syndrome and through local Down syndrome parent organizations. A lot of hope may come from the information parents learn about Down syndrome, such as the increasing life expectancy and the remarkable accomplishments of some individuals with Down syndrome. Even the stereotype that people with Down syndrome are always happy, affectionate, and socially outgoing can be encouraging, helping the new parent to form a positive new picture of the person their infant will become.

As time goes by, life may settle down into a new routine, a new normal. Life with a new baby is busy, but in many ways, it may not differ from life with any new baby as much as was first feared. Infancy gives way to toddlerhood, and before long, it is time to think about preschool. Often parents enjoy opportunities to connect with other parents of children with Down syndrome. But for some parents, these connections can add as much concern as they do comfort or companionship. Some parents notice that their children with Down syndrome don't seem to be doing the same things the other kids are doing. This can raise a lot of questions. Is my child okay? Is my child developing more slowly? Am I not doing what I should be doing as a parent? The observations leading to these questions can be vague, and so the concerns may be dismissed. But when the same questions are raised over and over, some parents experience a great deal of anxiety. For many parents, these questions and the anxiety they generate lead to the first suspicions about autism, although some parents report having had suspicions that began in infancy.

Common Emotions

The journey leading to the diagnosis of autism in children with Down syndrome can be very long and complicated. It is complicated by conflicting emotions, lack of information, professionals who may not be aware of the possibility of co-occurring diagnosis, and other factors. Because this journey can be so long and is different for every family, the emotions experienced when the diagnosis is finally reached can be very different. There is no roadmap to guide parents through this unexpected detour in raising their child. This might add confusion, but it also means that there is no right or wrong way to feel. All emotions experienced are valid and may provide clues to the steps the parent may take while adjusting to this unexpected turn.

Chronic Sorrow

Much has been written about the experiences of parents whose children have developmental disabilities, particularly their response to the diagnosis. Some of the information published is research-based, some theoretical, and some anecdotal. In general, however, there are two main ideas presented about this experience. The first is that parents have a grief reaction that progresses through various stages over time, eventually ending with a feeling of resolution. The specific stages outlined vary with the theory, but might include shock, despair, denial, guilt, withdrawal, acceptance, and adjustment, among other possibilities. The common theme is that at some point, this process is completed. The second significant idea, called chronic sorrow, was first described by Simon Olshansky in 1962. Briefly, the chronic sorrow theory is that parents will experience periods of time when the intense grieving reoccurs and that these periods may go on indefinitely. In other words, there is no real end point.

At this point, little has been published regarding the experience of parents whose children are diagnosed with a second developmental disability, so it is unclear whether either of these theories might describe the experience of parents of children with DS-ASD. However, based on the shared experiences of many parents, it is clear that parents experience a whole range of emotions when learning of this second diagnosis. These might include fear, anger, frustration, resentment, jealousy, relief, sadness, guilt, self-recrimination, disappointment, validation, isolation, loneliness, and probably others as well. These emotions may be experienced simultaneously or independently. They may be brief or long term; mild or intense.

Fear

When parents learn that their child has autism in addition to Down syndrome, they may experience fear of the unknown all over again, taking them back to the way they felt when they first learned of their child's Down syndrome diagnosis. There is so much to learn and the waters are mostly uncharted. Parents may have fears about their child's future needs and potential. They may feel fear and uncertainty about their ability to be a good parent to their child. They may fear the impact on their other children, on their marriage or partnerships, and on their financial stability. These fears may resolve with time, information, and support, or may persist indefinitely to varying degrees.

Anger/Frustration

Anger is commonly associated with the grieving process, and many parents grieve the autism diagnosis, so it is not surprising that anger is a common reaction in this situation. In addition to feeling anger that their child is affected, some parents are frustrated and angry that the professionals in their child's life didn't recognize the signs of autism sooner. Some parents have had to fight to find providers who will even consider this possibility and then may feel anger at the additional work and anguish they experienced. Some are angry that their child may have missed out on receiving targeted interventions sooner because of the delayed diagnosis. Others may feel anger that others do not see or believe in their child's ability to learn.

> *"I feel our biggest challenge is getting people to see [our daughter]— to see her potential and to challenge her, respect her, and believe in her. Too often people underestimate her before they have really given her a chance. This is very disheartening, especially when it is a 'professional.' I feel this is more detrimental to her than her actual disability."*

Resentment/Jealousy

It is not uncommon for parents to feel a certain resentment or even jealousy of parents whose children have Down syndrome but not autism. It is not that they wish more challenges on these other children or their parents, but instead feel the unfairness of their child's or their own burden. This is one reason some parents choose to withdraw from events or groups organized by Down syndrome organizations. The contrast in where their child is developmentally as compared to children without autism can be painful and can fuel this resentment.

Isolation

Parents of children with DS-ASD have often stated that they don't feel as if they quite fit within the Down syndrome community or the autism community. Instead, they feel that their child is significantly different than those in either group and that their own needs are also quite different. However, in many communities, there is no organization or group specifically for families of children with DS-ASD, so parents often feel a strong sense of isolation. Previous friendships may fade because of a sense that others can't quite understand their lives any more. Additionally, the needs of their children can be great enough that there is not enough time to devote to other relationships in their lives, leading to real loneliness. Some parents find support from local organizations, and others find support by connecting with parents of children with the co-occurring diagnosis through the Internet.

Disappointment

As mentioned above, when parents are initially adjusting to the diagnosis of Down syndrome, some find comfort or encouragement in the things they learn about children with Down syndrome, including the not-so-accurate but appealing idea that all children with Down syndrome are happy, affectionate, and loving. These characteristics can be true of some individuals with Down syndrome but certainly not all, and this holds true for those with DS-ASD as well. As parents of children with DS-ASD watch their children grow and develop, they may feel disappointment if their child doesn't display these expected characteristics, or if their child's development lags more than they expected.

Some parents also harbor a hope that their child might "outgrow" some autistic characteristics, and then feel disappointed if their child does not. They may also be disappointed if they try a treatment or therapy that is supposed to help children with Down syndrome or autism, but then it fails to produce the hoped-for changes.

Guilt

Just as many parents feel some guilt when they first learn that their child has Down syndrome, wondering if they might have done something to cause it, some parents feel guilt when they find out that their child also has autism. They may wonder whether anything they did or did not do might have caused or contributed to the autism. They may feel guilt that they were disappointed in their child's progress prior to learning that she has the added diagnosis of autism. They may feel guilt that they didn't see or seek the autism diagnosis sooner. As they learn about strategies and interventions to educate and support individuals with autism, they may feel guilt that they aren't able to do enough for their child. All of these possible sources of guilt may lead to self-recrimination as well.

These thoughts and feelings may be unavoidable to some extent, but when possible, it may be more helpful for parents to try to give themselves credit for all they have done and are doing for their family. I recommend that parents look toward what they can do in the future rather than focusing on what may have already occurred.

Relief

For some parents, finally confirming the diagnosis of autism may bring a sense of relief and validation. For parents who have long suspected autism or who have had a long journey to get to diagnosis, there may be a sense of relief that there really are answers to some of their questions. Some par-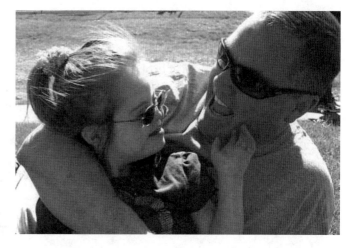ents express a sense of validation that their observations of their child's development were accurate and meaningful and that they were able to persevere in obtaining the professional evaluation needed. For many parents, getting the ASD label is a form of relief, since it provides an explanation for their child's behaviors and they can now "justify" to others that their child has additional challenges beyond Down syndrome.

For those who do feel relief and validation, this can provide the confidence needed to begin the next process—learning more about autism, particularly autism in individuals with Down syndrome.

The Kaleidoscope of Emotions

It is a rare parent in this situation who only feels one or two of these emotions or who only experiences them once. In most cases, parents will feel many of these feelings and will feel them more than once. Adjusting to something so unexpected in your child's life, and therefore your own life, doesn't happen all at once. Adjustment will be ongoing. Therefore, the feelings that are part of the process are likely to crop up again and again. It may be helpful to remember that your child is the same child as before the diagnosis. Getting that diagnosis didn't change the child. Instead, it gives you more information with which to proceed with the job of loving, teaching, and advocating for your child.

Relationships

Mother and Father

In some families, both parents may share in the concerns or the steps that led to the diagnosis of autism. In other families, however, one parent may be alone in this journey while the other either steps aside to watch and wait or openly disagrees with the decision to seek an evaluation and diagnosis.

In any case, once the diagnosis has been made, parents may experience different feelings than one another and at different times. This can add to the distress of the situation. However, it may be a comfort for parents to realize that having different reactions to this situation is probably more common than not. Even the closest relationships are made up of two people with different backgrounds and different experiences, so their response to the same situation won't necessarily be the same.

Having patience with one another and being willing to listen to thoughts and emotions that may be different from one's own may help a struggling couple be able to remain mutually supportive and focused on helping their child. Some may benefit from family counseling.

Grandparents and Extended Family

Grandparents and other extended family members may have their own thoughts and feelings about the additional diagnosis of autism, and these may not always match those of the parents. When this happens, conflicts can arise, causing added stress for all involved.

Family members may not be particularly well informed about autism, may suggest that the fault lies with poor parenting, or may suggest treatments that you, the parents, have already ruled out. If this occurs, you may try letting your extended family members know that you need their support and perhaps suggest some ways they can help. For example, you might ask your family members to explore some resources to help become more informed or give them specific tasks such as running errands.

If family members do not welcome the suggestions or are not able to provide the kind of support needed, you may have to limit the type or quantity of contact you have with family members who add more stress than support to your already challenging life.

Finding Support and Moving Forward

While parents of children with DS-ASD may sometimes feel alone in this experience, there are expanding efforts to make support and help available. There is a growing awareness of the needs of those with DS-ASD, and efforts are underway in different parts of the country to meet these needs. Those who find themselves struggling with their own emotions regarding the second diagnosis may benefit from working with a professional counselor such as a grief, marriage, or family counselor, psychologist, or a spiritual leader.

There are many reasons to remain hopeful about the future. Awareness about the co-occurring diagnosis of Down syndrome and autism is growing rapidly and with it, support. As more is learned about the intersection of Down syndrome and autism, better health and education strategies will likely become clearer, paving the way for brighter futures to come.

> *"We are in a more accepting place today. I don't see it as a black and white label anymore. Does she, doesn't she? It doesn't matter what the label is, it's just another piece of understanding (our child). I don't feel it's the worst thing in the world, but it certainly makes her life more challenging. I would take the autism piece away in a second. I know there are many parents who wouldn't change a thing even if they could (I try to channel this attitude), but it's hard to watch her struggle with her body awareness, communication, and social situations when she wants it so much . . . wanting to be accepted and included. She works very hard and we are so proud of her, the way she puts herself out there every day and has to work so hard just to pull everything together.*

> *Our kids are amazing!!! How can people see anything different? I often wonder—if our world were a more accepting, supportive place, if we could just be there for one another as a whole, to look out for one another—if a disability would in fact be a disability or just a difference?"*

Acknowledgment

I would like to acknowledge and thank the parents who have generously shared their time and experiences with me to help me grow in understanding and to pass along their valuable insight to others.

References

Capone, G.T. (Sept./Oct. 1999). Down syndrome and autistic spectrum disorder: A look at what we know. *Disability Solutions 3* (5-6).

Olshansky, S. (April 1962). Chronic sorrow: A response to having a mentally defective child. *Social Casework 43:* 190-95.

Searle, S. Jr. (April 1978). Stages of parent reaction: Mainstreaming. *Exceptional Parent* (April): 23-27.

Wikler, L., Wasow, M., & Hatfield, E. (Jan. 1981). Chronic sorrow revisited: Parent vs. professional depiction of parents of mentally retarded children. *American Journal of Orthopsychiatry:* 63-70.

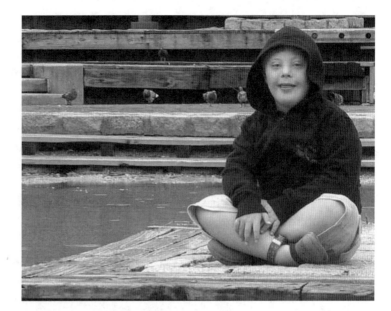

3

The Genetics of Down Syndrome and Autism Spectrum Disorder

Ellen Roy Elias, MD, FAAP, FACMG

Introduction

The prevalence of autism spectrum disorders (ASDs) is a topic of intense study. In 2003, pediatricians were shocked to see figures from the Centers for Disease Control (CDC) citing a prevalence of about 1:110 U.S. children (Yeargin-Allsopp, Karapurkar, et al., 2003). More recently reported figures suggest the prevalence of ASD may be as high as 110:10,000 (about 1:91) in the United States (Kogan et al., 2007). In children with Down syndrome, the prevalence is felt to be much higher—close to 1:10 (Hepburn et al., 2008).

Why do such a large number of children with DS have ASD, and why is this association about ten times as great as in the general population? The answer to this question is not currently known, but as the genetic causes of autism are becoming better understood, and the association of DS with ASD has become more obvious, this question has become of great research interest.

This chapter will explore common genetic causes of autism, and discuss possible genetic mechanisms that may be contributing to the association between DS and ASD.

Background: Is Autism Genetic?

There have been many epidemiologic studies which show that autism spectrum disorders have a clear underlying genetic cause. How do scientists know that a disorder is genetic? There are several clues that indicate that ASDs have an underlying genetic cause.

One important clue suggesting that a disorder has an underlying genetic cause is to study whether the disorder is familial, or occurs more often in family members (such as siblings) than expected by chance alone. There is clearly an increased risk of autism in siblings and family members. When one child in a family has autism, there is a 3 percent chance that his or her sibling will also have autism—which is about 100 times the prevalence of autism in the general population (Fombonne, 2003). This risk may be underestimated in families, because people who have a child with an ASD tend to limit family size, and people with autism tend not to reproduce.

Another important clue to the genetic nature of autism is to study the rate of autism in twins, comparing identical or monozygotic (MZ) twins—who have identical genetic makeup—to fraternal twins—who are genetically similar, as they are siblings, but do not have identical genes. If twins have the same presentation, this is called concordance. The concordance of autism in identical twins is much higher than in fraternal twins, as would be expected. Autism is about 300 times more common in a MZ co-twin than in the general population. However, the concordance rate is less than 100 percent. (That is, when one identical twin has autism, the other twin does not always have autism too.) This suggests that there are other, nongenetic factors that play a role.

A third clue that autism has an underlying genetic etiology is that autism is more common in males than in females. The male predominance is more pronounced in individuals in which autism is not associated with intellectual disabilities. In individuals with autism who have a normal IQ, the ratio is almost 6 males: 1 female. In individuals with autism who have a moderate to severe intellectual disability, the ratio is almost 2 males: 1 female. One explanation for this disparity may be that many genes causing autism lie on the X chromosome. Males, who have only one X chromosome, would manifest an abnormality if a gene on the X chromosome is mutated. Females, however, have two X chromosomes and are therefore less likely to show an effect of the same mutated gene. (Although one of a girl's X chromosomes is affected by a mutation, her other one may not be, and can therefore "override" the effects of the mutation.)

A fourth and important clue is the fact that many patients with known genetic disorders also have autism. In other words, a number of genetic disorders are clearly associated with, and felt to cause, autism. Some of the more common genetic disorders associated with autism are covered in the next part of this chapter.

Even though many clues point to the association between a genetic etiology and autism, it is still very difficult to determine a clear cause of autism for the majority of people with ASD (Schaefer & Mendelsohn, 2008; Johnson & Myers, 2007). There are several important reasons for this difficulty. First of all, there is not just one genetic cause, but actually thousands of different genes that are associated with autism. Thanks to the development of highly sophisticated genetic diagnostic tools, we are just beginning to be able to identify some of these genes. Secondly, there are other factors that affect inheritance, such as epigenetic factors, which will be explained later in this chapter. Epigenetic 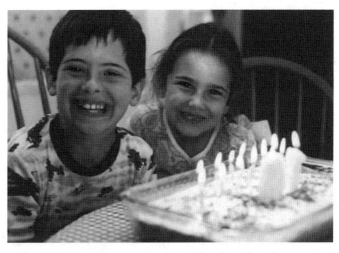 factors can complicate and affect certain genetic processes, and lead to developmental disabilities and autism. Thirdly, other factors, such as environmental influences (e.g., maternal alcohol consumption during pregnancy) (Abel & Hanningan, 2005), may in and of themselves be associated with autism, or may interact with other genetic and epigenetic factors and lead to autism.

Known Genetic Causes of Autism

As mentioned above, a number of genetic disorders are associated with autism. Examples of the most common ones are described below. Later in the chapter, there will be further discussion of whether testing for these disorders should be considered in a person with both Down syndrome and autism.

Chromosome Abnormalities

Any chromosomal abnormality associated with intellectual disability can also present with autistic features (Marshall et al., 2008). Whenever a chromosomal abnormality is associated with autism, this is exciting, as it may give a clue as to the location of autism candidate genes. Many of these chromosomal abnormalities associated with autism have been published, including genes on 1p, 2q, 7q, 13q, 16p, and 19q. (Chromosomes have a short arm called the p arm and a long arm called the q arm. So, 1p refers to genes on the short arm of the first chromosome; 19q refers to genes on the long arm of the 19th chromosome.)

In addition to Trisomy 21 (Down syndrome), other chromosome abnormalities that have a high rate of autism include Trisomy 13, and several different abnormalities involving the long arm of chromosome 15. (See the section below on epigenetic factors for a more detailed discussed of chromosome 15 abnormalities.)

A new technology called comparative genetic hybridization microarray allows the detection of extremely subtle DNA changes, including tiny pieces missing (deletions) or extra pieces (duplications or partial trisomies). This technology has allowed the diagnosis of chromosome abnormalities so subtle that they were completely missed with routine chromosome analysis. As this technology is used more and more in patients with autism, it is expected that new and additional autism candidate genes will emerge (Kidd et al., 2008; Glessner et al., 2009). Microarray is now routinely used as a first-line diagnostic test for children with the sole diagnosis of autism and is being investigated as a research tool in patients with both DS and autism.

Fragile X Syndrome

Fragile X syndrome is a common genetic disorder that is caused by a mutation in a gene called FMR1, located on the X chromosome (Hatton et al., 2006). About one-third of children with fragile X have autism, and about 2 to 6 percent of children diagnosed with autism have fragile X syndrome. People with fragile X syndrome have some characteristic features, including a relatively large head and a long face. Their joints may be hyperextensible. Males with fragile X can have enlargement of their testicles.

Rett Syndrome

Rett Syndrome (Lam et al., 2000) is a disorder that is seen almost exclusively in females, because the mutation is generally lethal in a male fetus. It is caused by a mutation in a gene called MECP2, located on the long arm of the X chromosome. Girls with Rett syndrome usually have a period of normal development during early infancy, but then start to lose milestones, and develop seizures. Often a characteristic hand wringing behavior develops. Autism is also common.

Rett syndrome is an important diagnosis to consider in girls and women with the combination of autism and seizures. The diagnosis is made by a specific blood test to analyze the MECP2 gene. (A chromosome analysis or microarray test would not detect this mutation.)

Epigenetic Mechanisms and Imprinting

Some people have genetic disorders that are caused not by changes in DNA, such as an extra piece or an altered gene, but changes in how the DNA code is being read by the body. These are called epigenetic mechanisms.

One particular epigenetic mechanism that is fairly well understood is called imprinting. With imprinted regions of DNA, certain genes are only read if they come from the chromosome that was inherited from the mother, and others only from the chromosome which came from the father. If an error in passing on DNA from the parent to the child occurs, then the child can manifest a genetic disorder that causes autism. Examples of such errors include:

- the child receives two copies of a chromosome from one parent and none from the other (called uniparental disomy),

- the DNA is mislabeled so that it looks like uniparental disomy has occurred,
- there is a missing or extra piece of DNA from one of these imprinted regions.

Epigenetic problems may be seen with increased frequency in children who were the product of pregnancies conceived via advanced reproductive technologies such as in vitro fertilization (IVF).

Angelman Syndrome and Abnormalities on Chromosome 15

Angelman syndrome (Clayton-Smith & Laan, 2003) is the best known of the disorders of the long arm of the 15th chromosome (15q). It affects the UBE3A gene derived from the mother. Children with Angelman syndrome have autism, severe intellectual disabilities, seizures, increased muscle tone in the lower extremities, and characteristic facial features. Angelman syndrome can occur in both boys and girls. Angelman syndrome can be caused by a deletion of the 15q inherited from the mother, which can be detected by microarray. It can also be caused by imprinting errors on chromosome 15, which require specialized DNA testing to detect.

There are other abnormalities on chromosome 15q that are associated with autism. These include having an extra piece of DNA, inherited from the mother, in the middle of 15q, or having an extra marker chromosome, which is made of pieces of chromosome 15q.

Metabolic Disorders

Inborn errors of metabolism are disorders in which an enzyme (protein) is missing or defective, leading to an inability of the body to perform a biochemical reaction that is necessary for normal functioning of the body and brain. There are many metabolic disorders associated with intellectual disabilities and autism. One example is *Smith-Lemli-Opitz syndrome,* a metabolic disorder caused by an inability of the body to make cholesterol (Sikora et al., 2006). Patients with the severe form of SLOS have unusual features and many birth defects in addition to severe intellectual disabilities and autism. Patients with the milder form of SLOS may only display autism and mild webbing of the second and third toes. The diagnosis of SLOS is confirmed by a special blood test looking for elevated levels of the compound called 7-dehydrocholesterol, which the body cannot turn into cholesterol.

Most inborn errors of metabolism are inherited as *autosomal recessive traits.* These are disorders that do not affect an individual unless he inherits the trait from both parents. If he only inherits the trait from one parent, he is a carrier and can pass the trait on to his own children, but does not have symptoms of the disorder himself. When both parents are carriers (carry a mutation in one of their genes) there is a 25 percent chance with each pregnancy that the baby might inherit this mutated gene from both parents. This class of disorders is seen with increased frequency if the parents are related to each other, or consanguineous.

Neurocutaneous Disorders

Neurocutaneous disorders are disorders which have both neurological/developmental symptoms and abnormal skin findings. Tuberous Sclerosis (Gutierrez, Smalley & Tanguay, 1998) is such a disorder. It causes white spots on the trunk and an acnelike rash on the face. People with TS often develop growths in the brain and kidney and have autistic features, and they usually have seizures and developmental delays.

Another common neurocutaneous disorder is Neurofibromatosis (NF) (Hersh & Committee on Genetics, 2008), which is associated with brown spots on the skin, freckles in the armpits and groin, and growths from neural tissues, including the brain, spinal cord, and other nerves. Most people with NF have normal cognitive abilities, but a minority have intellectual disabilities and autism.

Both TS and NF are passed on as autosomal dominant traits. That is, there is a 50:50 chance of passing on this condition from an affected parent to a child. In most children with TS and NF, the diagnosis is made based on observing the typical skin findings.

PTEN Mutations

A gene called PTEN (Marsh, Kum, Lunetta, et al., 1999), when mutated, causes a cancer-predisposition syndrome in adults called Cowden Syndrome (CS). Adults with CS are intellectually normal, but have a predisposition to developing malignancies, including breast cancer, thyroid cancer, and colon cancer, at an early age. This same gene mutation in a child can cause a disorder called Bannayan-Riley-Ruvalcaba syndrome, which results in autism and macrocephaly (a very large head circumference, greater than the 98th percentile). Boys with this condition can have unusual freckling on the penis.

It is important to test for PTEN mutations in children with autism and large heads, as the risk of cancer is increased in patients with PTEN mutations. Because this is a dominant disorder, if a child has a PTEN mutation, it is also important to test the parents to see if they might have CS and an increased cancer risk. This diagnosis is made by molecular testing of the PTEN gene in blood.

DNA Copy Number Variation

With the advent of new technology that allows us to see very subtle changes in DNA, we now understand that there is widespread variation in DNA called copy number variation (CNV), felt to affect about 0.4 percent of a person's DNA or genome. (That is, some individuals have fewer or more copies of a specific gene than other individuals do.)

By testing children with autism with this new technology (microarray), we have learned that copy number variation of certain genes is more common in patients with autism spectrum disorders. Many new genes that are believed to cause autism have been discovered in this way, including genes on chromosome 21. Because the microarray test can detect these subtle DNA changes, which were not detectable by older genetic testing methods, the microarray test has supplanted the traditional karyotype (chromosome) testing as the test of choice in children with developmental disabilities of unknown cause and autism.

What Causes the Association between Down Syndrome and Autism?

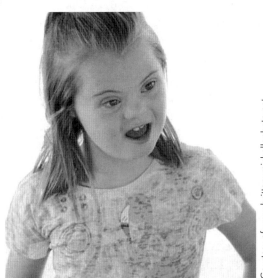

Courtesy of www.brittanymichellephoto.net

Given the many different known causes of autism listed above, and the knowledge that we have probably just begun to scratch the surface in our understanding of all the genetic etiologies contributing to autism, is it possible to better understand why so many people with DS also have autism? Yes. Although we do not definitively know all the reasons that autism is more common among people with Down syndrome, we are beginning to understand some of the connections. The answers to the questions below can better help parents understand why their child might have a dual diagnosis.

Are autism spectrum disorders associated with IQ and does this have a genetic basis?

It is true that many people with autism also have intellectual disabilities. It is also true that many individuals with more severe levels of intellectual disability also display features of autism. This is true not just for DS, but for many other genetic problems as well. Why certain people with DS learn at a faster rate, and why others have more significant cognitive disabilities and display features along the autism spectrum, is not well understood. It is possible that genetic factors that contribute to the rate of developmental progress and ultimate intellectual functioning may also be implicated in the presence of autism.

Is it possible that a child with DS also has another secondary diagnosis that is contributing to the autism?

For example, could a child have both DS and Fragile X, or both DS and Tuberous Sclerosis? Given how common autism spectrum disorders are now felt to be, this is certainly a possibility. However, to date there have been no large studies that have screened many children with both DS and ASD and tested for all of the common causes of ASD listed above. How many people with both DS and ASD also carry another diagnosis is therefore not known.

Should children with both DS and ASD be tested for other autism-causing conditions?

It is not unreasonable for a child with both DS and ASD to be evaluated by an experienced specialist such as a geneticist to determine whether additional diagnostic testing is appropriate. This is because: 1) many of the common causes of autism such as Fragile X syndrome are inherited in known genetic patterns that carry a high risk of recurrence in future pregnancies, or 2) have other implications for medical care, such as the increased cancer risk seen in PTEN mutations, or 3) have multiple medical issues such as are seen in SLOS.

For example, if the person has unusual skin lesions, one of the neurocutaneous disorders should be considered. If the person has an unusually large head and there is a strong family history of cancer at a young age, PTEN testing should be considered. If the family history suggests that individuals with autism are on the maternal side of the family, or the maternal grandfather has a Parkinson-like disorder, Fragile X testing should be considered. If the parents are distant relatives, and the child has webbing of the second and third toes, then SLOS should be considered. The decision to test for other disorders in addition to DS is one that should be made carefully, by an experienced clinician, based on the child's history and physical features, and the family history.

If Down syndrome is the sole diagnosis, what is it about having trisomy 21 that increases the risk of also having autism?

This is an intriguing question, the answer to which is not currently known. However, we may know the answer fairly soon, thanks to new genetic technology. As explained above, genetic studies have shown that copy number variation involving several genes on chromosome 21 have been associated with autism. The new genetic technologies make it possible to determine not only that a person has an extra copy of chromosome 21, but what the pattern of the DNA actually looks like on chromosome 21, especially of those genes that have been associated with autism in other patients. This technology is now being used on a research basis to compare the copy number variation that might be seen in a person with DS plus ASD, versus a person with DS and a more typical developmental course. Eventually, this should enable us to determine if there is a specific CNV pattern associated with autism.

It is also possible that there are other genes or proteins coded for by genes elsewhere on other chromosomes that are affected by the presence of trisomy 21, which may be causing the autism. With advances in sophisticated genetic technologies that study gene:gene and protein:protein interactions, it is now possible to look more closely at people with trisomy 21 and autism and try to understand whether there are certain DNA or protein findings that are unique to this group. These kinds of studies are tremendously exciting and offer great hope that we may one day better understand the underlying cause of autism in DS. However, they are still in their infancy.

In the near future, it will be possible for families to volunteer to participate in research protocols designed to answer these questions.

Conclusions

Autism spectrum disorders are incredibly common, occurring in about 1 out of 91 children in the United States. Children with Down syndrome are almost ten times as likely to also have autism, for reasons that are not clearly understood at this time.

There are many known genetic causes of autism, and advances in technology are allowing for the discovery of many new causes. The genetics of autism are complex (Pickler & Elias, 2009). We are just beginning to understand some of the many genetic mechanisms that can lead to intellectual disabilities and autism.

It is possible that a person with DS and ASD also carries a second, unrelated diagnosis that is contributing to the autistic features. The presence of other symptoms or physical features not common in DS, or a history of other individuals with autism in the family, may indicate the need for additional genetic testing.

It is believed that certain genes on chromosome 21 may confer an increased risk of autism. It is also possible that certain genes on chromosome 21 may interact with other genes on other chromosomes, contributing to an autism presentation. Sophisticated genetic studies are underway to study these possibilities further.

Further studies are clearly needed to investigate the association of DS and ASD, and help us better understand the causes of the high prevalence of this association. A better understanding may lead in the future to more effective treatments and interventions.

References

Abel, E.L. & Hanningan, J.H. (2005). Maternal risk factor in fetal alcohol syndrome: Provocative and permissive influences. *Neurotoxicology and Teratology 17*: 445.

Clayton-Smith, F. & Laan, L. (2003). Angelman syndrome: A review of the clinical and genetic aspects. *Journal of Medical Genetics 40:* 87-95.

Fombonne, E. (2003). Epidemiologic survey of autism and other pervasive developmental disorders. *Journal of Autism and Developmental Disorders 33:* 365-82.

Glessner, J.T. et al. (2009). Autism genome-wide copy number variation reveals ubiquitin and neuronal genes. *Nature 459):* 569-73.

Gutierrez, G.C., Smalley, S.L., & Tanguay, P.E. (1998). Autism in tuberous sclerosis complex. *Journal of Autism and Developmental Disorders 28:* 97-103.

Hatton, D.D. et al. (2006). Autistic behavior in children with fragile X syndrome: Prevalence, stability and the impact of FMRP. *American Journal of Medical Genetics A140 (17):* 1804-13.

Hepburn, S., Philofsky, A., Fidler, D., & Rogers, S. (2008). Autism symptoms in toddlers with Down Syndrome: A descriptive study. *Journal of Applied Research in Intellectual Disabilities 21(1):* 48-57.

Hersh, J.H. and the Committee on Genetics. (2008). Health Supervision for Children with Neurofibromatosis. *Pediatrics 21(3):* 633-42.

Johnson, C.P. & Myers, S.M. (2007). Identification and evaluation of children with autism spectrum disorders. *Pediatrics 120(5):* 1183.

Kidd, J.M. et al. (2008). Mapping and sequencing of structural variation from eight human genomes. *Nature 453:* 56-64.

Kogan, M.D. et al. (2009). Prevalence of parent-reported diagnosis of autism spectrum disorder among children in the US, 2007. *Pediatrics 124(4);* published online Oct 5, 2009.

Lam, C.W. et al. (2000). Spectrum of mutations in the MECP2 gene in patients with infantile autism and Rett syndrome. *Journal of Medical Genetics 37:* E41.

Marsh, D.J., Kum, J.B., Lunetta, K.L., et al. (1999). PTEN mutation spectrum and genotype-phenotype correlations in Bannayan-Riley-Ruvalcaba Syndrome suggest a single entity with Cowden Syndrome. *Human Molecular Genetics 8:* 1461-72.

Marshall, C.R. et al. (2008). Structural variation of chromosomes in autism spectrum disorders. *American Journal of Human Genetics 82(2):* 477-88.

Pickler, L.& Elias, E.R. (2009). The genetic evaluation of the child with autism spectrum disorders. In C. Johnson & S. Myers, eds. *Pediatric Annals. Autism Spectrum Disorders: What's New and What's to Do? 38(1):* 26-29.

Schaefer, G.B. & Mendelsohn, N.J. (2008). Genetics evaluation for the etiologic diagnosis of autism spectrum disorders. *Genetics in Medicine 10(1):* 4-12.

Sikora, D.M., Pettit-Kekel, K., Penfield, J., Merkens, L.S., & Steiner, R.D. (2006). The near universal presence of autism spectrum disorders in children with Smith-Lemli-Opitz Syndrome. *American Journal of Medical Genetics 140(14):* 1511-18.

Wolpert, C.M. et al. (2000). Three probands with autistic disorder and isodicentric Chromosome 15. *American Journal of Medical Genetics 96:* 365-72.

Yeargin-Allsopp, M. & Karapurkar, T., et al. (2003). Prevalence of autism in a U.S. metropolitan area. *Journal of the American Medical Association 289:* 49-55.

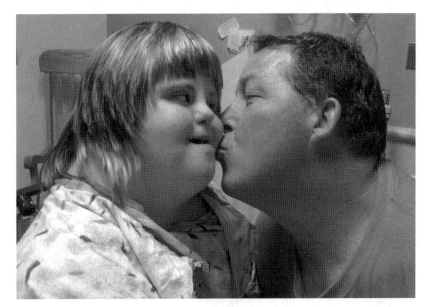

4

Medical Concerns in Individuals with DS-ASD

Fran Hickey, MD

The major challenge for families of children with Down syndrome (DS) who have symptoms consistent with autism spectrum disorder has been the persistent difficulty in receiving the proper diagnosis. The initial description of the dual diagnosis of Down syndrome and autism was reported in 1979 (Wakabayashi, 1979). This was supported by an excellent summary in the *Down Syndrome Quarterly* in 1985 (Coleman, 1986). However, although the dual diagnosis has been recognized in some quarters for over thirty years, there have been fewer than ten studies with fewer than seventy patients total described in the literature. Why is it still so difficult for many families to get a diagnosis?

This chapter will summarize the diagnostic dilemmas from a physician's point of view. In addition, the chapter will examine the most common medical problems experienced by people with a diagnosis of Down syndrome and autism, with an emphasis on how these problems differ from those who only have Down syndrome or autism.

Challenges in Diagnosis

One of the primary problems physicians encounter in diagnosing autism in children with autism is something called ***diagnostic overshadowing*** (Reiss, Levitan, &

Szyszko, 1982). This occurs when one diagnosis, such as Down syndrome, interferes with the detection of the other diagnosis because of the generalization that "those symptoms are just due to Down syndrome." This diagnostic overshadowing in Down syndrome interferes with the timely diagnosis of a variety of medical diagnoses, including gastro-esophageal reflux (GER), pneumonia, hypothyroidism, and even fractures. Often the underlying disability hampers the clinician's ability to come to the proper diagnosis. Likewise, when an individual is exhibiting symptoms of autism, the clinician may think the observed symptoms are due to delays caused by Down syndrome.

Besides diagnostic overshadowing, other challenges in the diagnosis of ASD in children with DS include intellectual disability, visual deficits, hearing deficits, sensory issues, and language delay. In children with DS, the delay in acquisition of language skills obviously adds to the diagnostic dilemma. This developmental language delay should be considered as a single entity. For example, if a child without Down syndrome is not speaking more than a couple words by the age of two, many parents and doctors might suspect autism. However, many children with Down syndrome, with and without autism, do not use speech to communicate at this age. These confounding variables mentioned above are not an explanation for social delays, lack of joint attention, stereotypical behavior, and other symptoms of ASD, however.

In 2007, the American Academy of Pediatrics (AAP) recommended routine screening of patients with Down syndrome for autism spectrum disorders (ASD) at 18 to 30 months (AAP, 2007). This was in part because the incidence of ASD in Down syndrome is high; at least 7 percent, according to some population-based studies (Kent, Evans, Moli, & Sharp, 1999; Hickey & Patterson, 2006). It is to be hoped that the AAP recommendation may result in more timely diagnosis of children who have autism in addition to DS. However, an accurate screening tool is not universally recognized for this high-risk population.

The delays in diagnosis and lack of recognition of developmental regression have affected the outcomes of patients with the DS-ASD dual diagnosis in a negative way. This chapter reviews the health considerations for children with Down syndrome and integrates the issues reported in children with autism spectrum disorders, with the hope that proper diagnosis of DS-ASD will lead to appropriate interventions.

Diagnostic Medical Challenges

The pediatrician or family practitioner has to recognize each child with Down syndrome as an individual and realize that any delays or symptoms are not "just Down syndrome." Assuming the child is involved in Early Intervention (EI) services, the physician needs to appreciate the concerns of the EI professionals regarding the child's loss of skills, lack of progress in language, or lack of socialization.

Reports from the ASD literature indicate that the age for presentation of autistic symptoms is between 15 and 18 months (Tuchman & Rapi, 1997) for children who do not have a dual diagnosis. Children with DS-ASD typically present with autistic concerns at a later age (Castillo et al., 2008). It is unclear if the delay in diagnosis is due to difficulties demarcating ASD characteristics from symptoms associated with Down syndrome, or if ASD occurs later in children with Down syndrome. Many anecdotal reports, however, indicate that parents of children with DS-ASD felt professionals had been dismissive of their concerns that their children with DS appeared to lack socialization skills, make insufficient communication progress, or lose skills.

The new autism identification directive from the AAP is that all children should be screened for autism from 18 months to 5 years. Healthcare providers and parents need to understand that most children with DS will fail the items testing language on these screens. However, children with DS will typically pass items dealing with socialization, play, and joint attention. Any social or interactive deficits are unusual in a child with DS and need to be addressed with further evaluation. As with all children, if there is any concern about autism by a family member, teacher, or professional, these concerns dictate a referral to a professional with expertise in autism.

The diagnostic team ideally should include a physician, a speech therapist, and a psychologist. The evaluation should include autism-specific diagnostic questionnaires along with ASD-specific tools such as the Autism Diagnostic Observation Schedule (ADOS) (Starr et al., 2005) and the Autism Diagnostic Interview-Revised (ADIR). However access to some of these assessments [ADOS and ADI-R] is often limited to a children's hospital or autism diagnostic center.

In screening children with DS for symptoms of ASD, it is important to bear in mind that there is a subset of children with DS who have a developmental and/or language regression as their presentation of autism. Approximately 20 to 30 percent of children whose sole diagnosis is ASD regress developmentally between 18-30 months (Tuchman & Rapin, 1997; Molloy et al., 2009). That is, there is a deterioration or loss of ability in a previously acquired skill in language, communication, or social skills. In individuals with DS-ASD, regression is reported to occur in 50 percent of the children. The age of regression in DS-ASD is significantly later than that reported in children with autism alone. One study (Castillo et al., 2008) found the average age in children with DS-ASD is 61 months—about 5 years.

This delayed onset of regressive symptoms in development in children with DS-ASD makes this diagnosis that much more difficult. The physician needs to realize that regression in DS is later and hence the onset of autistic symptoms is later. This is why yearly questions regarding social, adaptive, and language functioning are essential for children with Down syndrome, and a serial Modified Checklist for Autism in Toddlers (M-CHAT) may be useful. Obviously, an early diagnosis of ASD benefits the child so that proper interventions for ASD can be implemented.

The AAP's Medical Guidelines for Children with Down syndrome

To assist pediatricians in preventative medical care for children with Down syndrome, the American Academy of Pediatrics (AAP) has published guidelines for the health care of these children. Medically relevant guidelines will be reviewed in this chapter.

Medical Work-up for DS-ASD

After a child or adult with DS is initially diagnosed with ASD, he or she should receive a thorough medical work-up. The initial work-up should consider the increased medical risks associated with Down syndrome along with the ASD considerations. These pertinent DS medical issues include seizures, celiac disease, obstructive sleep apnea (OSA), and hearing and visual deficits. A combined DS-ASD evaluation includes:

- audiological (hearing) evaluations
- ophthalmological (vision) evaluations
- a lead test
- complete blood count
- iron studies
- liver function tests
- an electroencephalogram (EEG), depending on the medical/developmental history. This is because the seizure rate in DS is approximately 7 percent (Goldberg-Stern et al., 2001) and the reported seizure rate in ASD ranges from 7 to 30 percent (Barbaresi, Katusic, & Voigt, 2006).

Gastrointestinal System

Gastrointestinal symptoms are prevalent in Down syndrome. Initially, some children with DS have surgical emergencies with the presentation of Hirschsprung's or duodenal anomalies, including atresia or webs. The physician needs to be aware of

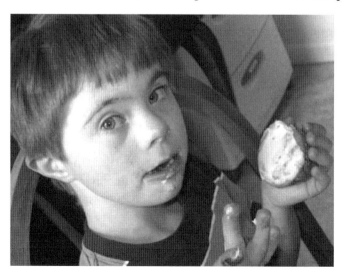

these comorbidities and keep a high index of suspicion. An infant with Down syndrome who has persistent vomiting needs an abdominal x-ray and should be strongly considered for an upper GI. Similarly, no stool passing in the first 24 hours of life indicates the need for an evaluation such as a rectal biopsy for Hirschsprung's disease.

In individuals with ASD, functional gastrointestinal symptoms are extremely common. (A GI problem is considered "functional" when no medical cause is found for it.) **Constipation** is the most widespread functional GI symptom, occurring in more than 30 percent of those who have ASD. **Food selectivity** (a limited repertoire of food) occurs in 25 of individuals with ASD. Most children with DS-ASD will have an increased predilection for constipation and abdominal pain. Often an abdominal x-ray is the only way to diagnose significant constipation, or, after treatment, to document evacuation of excessive stool. A consult with a dietitian may be beneficial to counsel the family about parameters for adequate nutrition.

Most studies show that *celiac disease* occurs in about 7 to 10 percent of children with Down syndrome (Book et al., 2001). The current recommendation is to screen for celiac disease at two or three years of age for children with Down syndrome; however, this guideline is currently under review by the AAP. Repeat testing for celiac disease has not been studied, but many Down syndrome clinics retest every three to four years.

Pediatric GI specialists (Hill et al., 2005) have recommended Human Leukocyte Antigen (HLA) testing and celiac testing in individuals such as those with Down syndrome who are at high risk for celiac disease. *Anti-tissue Transglutaminase Antibody (TTG-IgA)* and *IgA Antibody* are the recommended screening blood tests; positive tests are confirmed with biopsy by a gastroenterologist. This HLA testing provides information on genetic predisposition for celiac disease. If a high-risk child (such as one with DS) does not have this at-risk genetic finding [40 percent of the total population] then she would not need retesting. The other 60 percent of children with DS require retesting due to their genetic HLA predisposition to celiac disease.

Another reason this testing is relevant is because children with ASD have been reported to have difficulties with *dietary gluten* even without the diagnosis of celiac disease. Anecdotal cases include a child with ASD who improved significantly on a gluten-free diet (GFD) (Vaknin et al., 2004). Large controlled studies with children with ASD, however, have not shown that the gluten-free diet (GFD) improves GI difficulties or autistic symptoms (Millward et al., 2008). The medical community strongly recommends that children have a proven diagnosis of celiac disease prior to starting a lifelong gluten-free diet. GI specialists, dietitians, and nutritionists alike express concerns in using a GFD unnecessarily.

Gastroesophageal reflux (GER) has historically been reported as occurring more often in children with Down syndrome. Recent studies (Macchini, 2011) have noted an even more remarkable incidence of GER associated with DS. This implies that this disorder has been significantly underestimated in children with DS. In contrast, clinical studies concerning GER in individuals with ASD have noted no significant incidence.

Children with DS-ASD need close monitoring for GER since they are at risk medically and often lack communication skills to express discomfort and pain. GER needs to be considered in younger children also, because the GER may lead to silent aspiration. In turn, silent aspiration may lead to recurrent pneumonias and/or hypoxia, which subsequently can lead to pulmonary hypertension. Eventually the pulmonary hypertension may result in cor pulmonale, or irreversible pulmonary hypertension. Physicians need to strongly consider silent aspiration in individuals with DS-ASD, and should obtain a feeding evaluation if there is any feeding concern or unexplained pulmonary disease.

Pulmonary Problems

In the medical guidelines for children with Down syndrome (AAP, 2001), the only pulmonary medical problem screened for is *obstructive sleep apnea (OSA),* which is discussed below in the section on Sleep Concerns.

The other respiratory issue mentioned in the guidelines is the increased suscep-tibility to *respiratory infections.* Children with Down syndrome have many physical and genetic anomalies that put them at risk for airway and respiratory disease. Respi-ratory infections are responsible for approximately 80 percent of hospitalizations and ICU admissions in children with DS [McDowell & Craven, 1991]. The causes of the re-spiratory illnesses in Down syndrome are multifocal. In contrast, the only issue noted to be associated with respiratory illnesses in ASD is the possibility of immune defects.

Screening Blood Tests

ASD literature (Barbaresi, Katusic, & Voigt, 2006) suggests iron studies when children are being initially screened for an autism spectrum disorder. There is no re-port of a verified increase of anemia in individuals with ASD. However, *anemia* may occur due a nutritional deficiency that needs monitoring. In children with Down syn-drome, a recent study (Dixon et al., 2010) demonstrated the incidence of iron defi-ciency was 10 percent. Since the Complete Blood Count (CBC) indices are usually in-creased in Down syndrome, additional tests, including reticulocyte count, transferrin, and serum ferritin, are recommended.

As discussed previously, it is also recommended that children with DS-ASD be screened with an Anti-tissue Transglutaminase Antibody (TTG) and IgA Antibody. If the results are negative, the child needs retesting with a TTG every three years. If the TTG is elevated and concerning for celiac disease, the child should be referred to a pediatric GI specialist.

Sleep Concerns

Sleep concerns have been frequently reported in both children with Down syn-drome and children with ASD (see Chapter 9). Many of these sleep issues are related to behavioral sleep issues and other challenges. This sleep discussion will concentrate on the obstructive sleep apnea [OSA] issues that are common in DS, but not in ASD.

The incidence of OSA in those with DS is approximately 50 to 70 percent. The AAP medical guidelines therefore recommend that children with DS have a sleep study by 4 years of age to rule out obstructive sleep apnea.

A sleep study must be considered strongly in a differential diagnosis of the child presenting with autistic symptoms, whether or not she has symptoms of sleep apnea. In addition, a Sleep EEG should be added if there is a history of developmental regres-sion. See Chapter 9 for more information about sleep apnea and other sleep problems in children with DS-ASD.

Immune System

Immune deficits have been indicated in individuals with DS for decades; however, only a few studies have identified some of the deficits. Recurrent infections have a major impact on morbidity and mortality in DS, as recently described in otolaryngology (ear, nose, and throat) and pulmonology (Marcus et al., 1991; Shott et al., 2006). Common ENT issues for children with DS include frequent otitis media and subsequent hearing loss. Also, a tonsillectomy and adenoidectomy (T/A) is often recommended for treatment of upper airway obstruction, obstructive sleep apnea, or chronic tonsillitis in children with DS. In addition, pneumonia may occur repeatedly and lead to pulmonary hypertension and the need for supplemental oxygen.

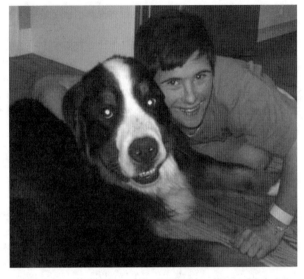

Studies have found that children with DS have a decrease in the number of lymphocytes (white blood cells that fight infection). Viral illnesses further exacerbate the children's relative lymphocytopenia (low white blood cells). Reductions in subpopulations of lymphocytes (CD4 T cells) have been identified (De Hingh et al., 2005) and are thought to play a role in the increased susceptibility of individuals with DS to Streptococcus pneumoniae and Hemophilus influenzae lung infections. It is speculated that impaired pulmonary immunological defenses may be related to decreases in IgG subclasses 4 and 2, which can be associated with recurrent illnesses, but there has been no direct clinical correlation demonstrated in patients with DS so far in the literature.

Due to this susceptibility to infection, it is important that children with Down syndrome receive all immunizations recommended by the American Academy of Pediatrics. In addition, for children with DS and chronic cardiac or pulmonary disease, the 23-valent pneumococcal polysaccharide vaccine (PPS23) is recommended at 2 years of age.

Summary

Children with Down syndrome and ASD are a specific population that warrants in-depth clinical research and funding to elucidate information regarding ASD that may benefit all children with ASD. Medical outreach is necessary to educate physicians and other professionals that these diagnoses coexist and that children with Down syndrome require the same developmental screening as all children.

References

AAP Committee on Genetics. (2001). Health supervision for children with Down syndrome. *Pediatrics 107(2):* 442-49.

American Academy of Pediatrics. (2007). AAP recommends autism screening for all infants. American Academy of Pediatrics 2007 National Conference and Exhibition. Presented October 29, 2007.

Barbaresi, W.J., Katusic, S.K., & Voigt, R.G. (2006). Autism: A review of the state of the science for pediatric primary health care clinicians. *Archives of Pediatrics & Adolescent Medicine 160(11):* 1167-75.

Book, L., Hart, A., Black, J., Fool, M., Zone, J.J., & Neuhausen, S.L. Prevalence and clinical characteristics of celiac disease in Down syndrome in a U.S. study. (2001). *American Journal of Medical Genetics 98(1):* 70-74.

Castillo, H., Patterson, B., Hickey, F., Kinsman, A., Howard, J.M., Mitchell, T., & Molloy, C.A. (2008). Difference in age at regression in children with autism with and without Down syndrome. *Journal of Developmental & Behavioral Pediatrics 29(2):* 89-93.

Coleman, M. (1986). Down's syndrome children with autistic features. *Down's Syndrome Papers and Abstracts for Professionals 9(3):* 1-2.

de Hingh, Y.C., van der Vossen, P.W., Gemen, E.F., Mulder, A.B., Hop, W.C., Brus, F., & de Vries, E. (2005). Intrinsic abnormalities of lymphocyte counts in children with Down syndrome. *Journal of Pediatrics 147(6):* 744-47.

Dixon, N.E., Crissman, B.G., Smith, P.B., Zimmerman, S.A., Worley, G., & Kishnani, P.S. (2010). Prevalence of iron deficiency in children with Down syndrome. *Journal of Pediatrics 157(6):* 967-71.

Goldberg-Stern, H., Strawsburg, R.H., Patterson, B., Hickey, F., Bare, M., Gadoth, N., et al. (2001). Seizure frequency and characteristics in children with Down syndrome. *Brain Development 23(6):* 375-78.

Hickey, F. & Patterson, B. (2006). Dual diagnosis of Down syndrome and autism. *International Journal on Disability and Human Development 5(4):* 365-68.

Hill, I.D., Dirks, M.H., Liptak, G.S., Colletti, R.B., Fasano, A., Guandalini, S., Hoffenberg, E.J., Horvath, K., Murray, J.A., Pivor, M., & Seidman, E.G.; North American Society for Pediatric Gastroenterology, Hepatology and Nutrition. (2005). Guideline for the diagnosis and treatment of celiac disease in children: Recommendations of the North American Society for Pediatric Gastroenterology, Hepatology and Nutrition. *Journal of Pediatric Gastroenterology and Nutrition 40(1):* 1-19.

Johnson, C.P., Myers, S.M., & the Council on Children with Disabilities. (2007). Identification and evaluation of children with autism spectrum disorders. *Pediatrics 120(7):* 1183-1215.

Kent, L., Evans, J., Moli, P., & Sharp M. (1999). Comorbidity of autistic spectrum disorders in children with Down Syndrome. *Developmental Medicine and Child Neurology 41:* 153-58.

Kusters, M.A., Verstegen, R.H., Gemen, E.F., & de Vries, E. (2009). Intrinsic defect of the immune system in children with Down syndrome: A review. *Clinical & Experimental Immunology156(2):* 189-93.

Macchini, F., Leva, E., Torricelli, M., & Valadè, A. (2011). Treating acid reflux disease in patients with Down syndrome: Pharmacological and physiological approaches. *Clinical and Experimental Gastroenterology 4:* 19-22.

Marcus, C.L., Keens, T.G., Bautista, D.B., von Pechmann, W.S., & Ward, S.L. (1991). Obstructive sleep apnea in children with Down syndrome. *Pediatrics 88(1):* 132.

McDowell, K.M. & Craven, D.I. (2011). Pulmonary complications of Down syndrome during childhood. *Journal of Pediatrics 158:* 319-25.

Millward, C., Ferriter, M., Calver, S., & Connell-Jones, G. (2008). Gluten- and casein-free diets for autistic spectrum disorder. *Cochrane Database of Systematic Reviews 2:* CD003498.

Molloy, C.A., Murray, D.S., Kinsman, A., Castillo, H., Mitchell, T., Hickey, F.J., & Patterson B. (2009). Differences in the clinical presentation of Trisomy 21 with and without autism. *Journal of Intellectual Disability Research 53 (Part 2):*143–51.

Reiss, S., Levitan, G.W., & Szyszko, J. (1982). Emotional disturbance and mental retardation: Diagnostic overshadowing. *American Journal of Mental Deficiency 86(6):* 567-74.

Shott, S.R., Amin, R., Chini, B., Heubi, C., Hotze, S., & Akers, R. (2006). Obstructive sleep apnea: Should all children with Down syndrome be tested? *Archives of Otolaryngology – Head & Neck Surgery 132(4):* 432.

Starr, E.M., Berument, S.K., Tomlins, M., Papanikolaou, K., & Rutter, M. (2005). Brief report: Autism in individuals with Down syndrome. *Journal of Autism and Developmental Disorders 35(5):* 665-73.

Tuchman, R. & Rapin, I. (1997). Regression in pervasive developmental disorders: Seizures and epileptiform electroencephalogram correlates. *Pediatrics 99:* 560-66.

Vaknin, A., Eliakim, R., Ackerman, Z., & Steiner, I. (2004). Neurological abnormalities associated with celiac disease. *Journal of Neurology 251(11):* 1393-97.

Wakabayashi, I. (1979) A case of infantile autism associated with Down's syndrome. *Journal of Autism and Developmental Disorders 9:* 31-36.

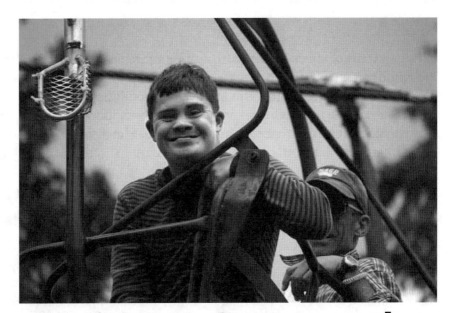

5

When Autism Is Suspected for Teens and Adults with Down Syndrome

Dennis E. McGuire, Ph.D., Elina R. Manghi, PsyD, LMFT, & Brian Chicoine, MD

One common concern voiced by families and caregivers who attend the Adult Down Syndrome Center of Lutheran General Hospital (ADSC) is that the behavior or characteristics of their family member with DS is an indication of an autism spectrum disorder (ASD). Because of the work of pioneering clinicians and researchers in the field, there is much better awareness among professionals and caregivers that ASD can coexist with Down syndrome (DS) (Capone, 1999; Reilly, 2009). Over the past ten years or more, there have been presentations on this topic at national conferences, and children with DS-ASD are now far more likely to be diagnosed with this condition than in the past. Still, there is a great deal of overlap in the descriptions and behavior of both DS and autism and it is not always clear to parents or professionals how the two syndromes differ.

These issues are particularly confusing to parents of people with DS who are in their late teen and adult years. For many of these families, there was little information and awareness of DS-ASD while their children were growing up. In fact, many parents who had concerns have reported that they could not find professionals who could help them, or they were told that ASD did not occur in people with DS.

This chapter will look at the behavior and characteristics of ASD and DS in teens and adults in order to help caregivers and professionals to better differentiate whether autism is a true concern. We will also discuss strategies to use when ASD is diagnosed. We will draw upon our experience in the ADSC to discuss these issues but we were also able to elicit the assistance of a colleague, Dr. Elina Manghi, to help us write this chapter. The late Dr. Manghi was a psychologist by training and an expert on ASD, and she had extensive experience with ASD and DS. She also added a key component to this chapter with her discussion of the complex art and science of the diagnosis of ASD.

Findings of the Adult Down Syndrome Center

At the ADSC, we serve the health and psychosocial needs of individuals with DS who are twelve years of age and older. Our purpose will be to describe what we have observed and documented for the patients at our center who show symptoms and behaviors of ASD, and also to compare them with same-age peers with DS who do not have ASD. We will limit our sample to individuals who are younger than 30 to have some uniformity in the sample, but also because the idea that ASD could coexist in DS has only been more widely accepted in the past ten to fifteen years. We have reviewed case records and have followed up with interviews of twenty-six individuals who were diagnosed with DS-ASD or who we believe have ASD because of symptoms and behaviors. We will also discuss how to differentiate DS-ASD from DS, how to diagnose ASD in this population, and what treatment strategies are effective when DS-ASD is found.

Parent Recollection of Childhood History

We will briefly discuss a general childhood history of individuals in our sample based on parental interviews and available records. There are some obvious inaccuracies and omissions in the parental interviews because they are based on a recollection of events that occurred between five to eighteen years in the past. Still, parental reports are quite consistent for individuals in the sample. It is interesting to note, too, that many families recalled painful experiences in the past. Most commonly, these painful experiences were due to critical or negative comments from family or friends, but also from teachers, staff, neighbors, and even strangers.

Parents clearly interpreted these criticisms to imply that if they were better parents, their child's problems would go away. Many parents also reported at least one incident in public settings where strangers accused them of being bad or abusive parents when their child displayed a tantrum or problem behavior. On the other hand, many of these same parents remembered other family, friends, teachers, staff, and professionals who took the time to understand and support them and their child despite whatever behavior the child displayed. These individuals made life far more tolerable for them.

Two Categories

Most families' descriptions of their child's history fit into one of two categories, which are similar to categories reported by Dr. George Capone (1999). In the first category, the child displayed autistic symptoms and behaviors from very early in child-hood and the families do not recall this as a result of a regression. In the second cat-egory, the child was reported to have had a major regression of previously mastered skills. Parents reported that the age of regression tended to be older, from 3 to 8 years, compared to the age of 2 to 3 years reported in the general population (who developed ASD). The later date of regression may be due to a delay in development for children with DS compared to the general population.

Of those families reporting a regression, some reported the type of severe and dra-matic regression similar to what Joan Medlen (1999) described so eloquently in her article "More than Down Syndrome: A Parent's View." For example, many children had verbal language, were social with caregivers and peers, and had creative play and other skills, before seemingly losing all these skills in a regression. Other parents, however, described a major regression, but also observed some differences in their sons and daughters even before the regression. Many noted there were differences in their child's response to them or to other children compared to other children with DS. They also frequently noted more fussiness and irritability, the presence of stereotypic behaviors (such as rocking and hand flapping), and a greater sensitivity to sensory stimuli (such as to touch, light, or sounds), as well as eating and sleeping difficulties. Thus, for many individuals in the sample, the distinction between first and second categories appears to be less clear or obvious.

Symptoms and Behaviors of ASD

Regardless of which category, described above, best described a child, the follow-ing symptoms and behaviors were reported by families in the sample:

Difficulties with Social Skills. Most notably, there was significant lack of social response or relatedness with family or friends. Parents also noted a definite lack of interest or ability in developing relationships with peers. Many children were antiso-cial, anxious, or fearful in the presence of people they did not know, even when they encountered visitors in their own home.

In the literature, individuals with DS-ASD have been reported to be a little more social than those with ASD without DS, and this was also reported by parents in our sample (Capone, 1999). Despite this, we found there is still a significant difference in social relatedness between individuals with DS-ASD and those with "just DS," as we will discuss at some length later in this chapter.

Difficulties in Communication. Most families in the second category (described above) reported a total loss of verbal communication as a result of a regression, but many children in the first category, who did not have a major regression, also had sig-nificant expressive language limitations, and quite a few were nonverbal.

Repetitive Behaviors. In both groups, most individuals developed or intensified stereotypic and repetitive motor behaviors such as hand flapping, spinning, or rock-ing. Many also developed an obsession or fascination with inanimate objects such as strings, lights, fans, mirrors, hands, fingers, and water. Many also lost the ability or interest in creative play, preferring instead to manipulate objects (often repetitiously) in rigid ways, such as lining up toys or other objects in fixed positions.

Typical Signs of ASD in Teens and Adults with Down Syndrome

- Significant lack of social response or relatedness with family or friends
- Lack of interest in or ability to develop relationships with peers
- Antisocial, anxious, or fearful in the presence of people they do not know
- For some, a history of regression, with loss of verbal communication
- If no regression, significant expressive language limitations or nonverbal
- Intensified stereotypic and repetitive motor behaviors (e.g., hand flapping, spinning, or rocking)
- Obsession or fascination with inanimate objects such as strings, lights, fans, mirrors, hands, fingers, and water
- Lack of ability or interest in creative play
- Manipulation of objects in rigid ways, such as lining up toys or other objects in fixed positions
- Intensified sensitivity to certain types of sensory input (hearing, touch, taste, smell, sight)
- Frequent tantrums and outburst, as well as verbal and physical aggression
- Great difficult in adjusting to transitions
- Dropping to the ground and refusing to move—a common strategy when refusing to respond to a change
- A little more social than those with ASD without DS

Sensory Issues. Many children also developed or intensified sensitivity to certain sensory inputs, such as hearing, touch, taste, smell, sight, and less-known body senses.

Behavioral Challenges. Parents also remember that their children had behavioral challenges, including frequent tantrums and outbursts, as well as verbal and physical aggression. Many parents also noted great difficulty in adjusting to transitions and that a common strategy when refusing to respond to a change was to drop to the ground and refuse to move. This is a particularly difficult strategy to counter because the person's body becomes dead weight. Families universally dread this behavior. Many had a name for it such as a "melt down" or a "drop and flop."

Current History for the Sample

ASD is a spectrum, and there were some significant differences in the intensity or severity of symptoms for individuals in the sample. Still, all of the people in our sample showed the core features of ASD. We can, however, make one important distinction between sample members based on how or when they were diagnosed or identified as having an autism spectrum disorder.

The first group was diagnosed with ASD in childhood, by a reputable diagnostician. Still, many of the parents in this group reported that they had problems locating a professional to diagnose their child.

A second group was not formally diagnosed by a trained psychologist or diagnostician, but they were told by someone who worked in some professional capacity that their child probably had an ASD, and this person had extensive contact with their son or daughter. Many times, parents respected the opinion of this person or professional. Many of these parents followed up with their own review of the literature (on autism and DS-ASD) and were knowledgeable about the issues. Families in this group gave a number of reasons why they did not seek a formal diagnosis. Some reported that they simply could not find a practitioner or a center that diagnosed ASD and DS, some could not afford an evaluation, others reported that they felt no need because they already knew, and still others reported they simply didn't find the time because of the demands of raising their child with DS-ASD.

A third group of individuals was also not diagnosed with ASD prior to coming to the ADSC. Families in this group clearly had grave concerns that something was wrong, and some even suspected autism (given what they had heard of the disorder), but they were not able to find a practitioner or any reputable source to help them give a name to their concerns.

Mental Health Diagnosis and Treatments

Despite the differences in when or how individuals were diagnosed, there was one major similarity for all groups. Most were diagnosed and treated by a variety of other mental health practitioners and were given a variety of other mental health diagnoses. Even families in the first group were quite often given other diagnoses and a host of treatments before finding the "right" diagnostician to identify the autism.

The most common of the diagnoses given by these practitioners included Attention Deficit Disorder, Oppositional Defiant Disorder, Obsessive Compulsive Disorder, Bipolar Disorder, Impulse Control Disorder, and Atypical Psychosis. The psychotropic medications prescribed included those that were the norm for treatment of these disorders, including the atypical antipsychotics, antidepressants, and mood stabilizers. Families reported that some of these treatments helped, while others did not. Quite a few of the families reported at least some problems with side effects associated with these medications, including most commonly weight gain, followed by agitation and sedation.

It is interesting to note that many parents, across all the groups, were told by medical and mental health practitioners that people with DS could not have ASD.

Current Problems and Issues Identified at the Center

As mentioned previously, at the Adult Down Syndrome Center, we serve the health and psychosocial needs of individuals with DS who are twelve years of age and older. Thus, individuals were seen at the Center five to eighteen years after parents first noted changes in their children. Regardless of which of the above three categories families were in, most reported that whatever positive strategies they learned to help support their child's development and behavior in childhood were often undermined by the developmental, physical, and environmental changes and challenges in the teen and adult years. These changes and challenges tended to create more extreme and unmanageable levels of stress. We found that most individuals with DS-ASD in our sample simply had too many stressors and vulnerabilities to come through the teen and adult years without experiencing major problems.

Stressors and Vulnerabilities

Like all individuals with DS, the people in the sample were at greater risk for a host of **health issues,** such as hypothyroid disorder, sleep apnea, GI problems, and celiac disease (inability to process gluten)—all of which may have a profound effect on the person's physical and mental well-being (Chicoine & McGuire, 2010). Additionally, sleeping and eating difficulties, as well as bowel and bladder issues, continued well beyond childhood for many people in the sample, creating enormous stress for parents, as well as for their son or daughter. For example, aside from sleep apnea (diagnosed in four individuals in the sample) many in our sample tended to have agitation as a result of stress in their lives. This agitation would continue well into the night-time hours, affecting their own and their parents' sleep. Over time, the detrimental effect on the family and person with DS increased as the sleep problems and sleep deprivation continued.

Hormonal changes were also a major cause of stress for teens and for parents in our sample. In our Center population, we found that hormonal changes for people with DS (with and without ASD) occurred close to or just a little after the age that people in the general population experienced them (McGuire & Chicoine, 2006). Adolescence brings on major physical changes in the body, such as the growth of body hair, the need for deodorant, the maturation of genitalia, and the onset of menses in women and nocturnal emissions in men. The latter two changes were understandably most disturbing to teens with DS-ASD.

Accompanying these hormonal changes are the notorious *fluctuations in mood* that are the hallmark of adolescence. This is a difficult and tumultuous period for people without intellectual disabilities. We found similarities in mood and behavior for adolescents with DS and those in the general population, but for teens with DS-ASD, the effect was even more intense and disruptive. No doubt the effect of hormonal changes were increased by communication difficulties that made it far more difficult for parents, teachers, or professionals to explain to individuals with DS-ASD what was happening to their bodies. Even parents who had other teenagers and who were prepared for a rocky road were surprised by the intensity and severity of mood and behavior fluctuations. Families reported a marked increase in anxiety and agitation, temper tantrums, oppositional behavior, rigid compulsions, and refusals to do just about anything.

For a number of individuals, there were other ***problems in public settings.*** For example, many in our sample often refused to use public toilets, which greatly limited activities in the community. For others, using a public toilet could too easily create trauma, which affected all elimination behavior.

Eating problems also continued to be a concern in teen and adult years. Many individuals were fussy eaters or had peculiar tastes, habits, or rituals when eating. Often, odd eating habits were precipitated by sensory issues, such as having an aversion to certain textures, smells, or sensations when eating. Whatever the cause of the eating habits or issues, the effect for many families was to create stress and a battleground at meals, particularly if the person's food choices were unreasonable or unhealthy.

In our Center, in general, we have found that many teens and adults with DS are susceptible to ***sensory problems,*** such as vision, hearing, and touch. These issues appear to be far more common and intense for people with DS-ASD and to interfere with their ability to go freely into the community. These individuals often find sensory stimuli such as lights, noises, large spaces, or crowds quite aversive.

Social Relatedness Issues

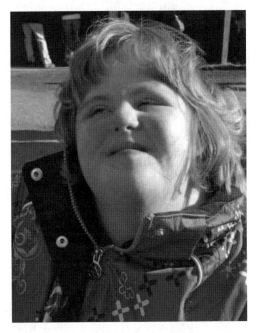

Perhaps the most important area of stress and vulnerability for the people in our sample was social skills and social relatedness. This is also the one key area that is different for persons with DS-ASD versus individuals with DS (as we will discuss at some length later). We live in a social world; thus, our ability to deal with others may have a profound effect on all areas of our life.

Most people with DS have an ability to engage others because of good social skills. This ability to interact may go a long way toward instilling goodwill and assistance from others, especially when experiencing problems or in times of need. In contrast, people with DS-ASD do not have this social ability. As a result, the lack of a smile or attempt to reach out to others may too easily result in a lack of understanding, patience, and sensitivity from others—in schools, recreation centers, extended family, and community settings. The families found that their children's problems with social skills often made it so much more difficult to get help and support when needed or to resolve issues when they occurred.

Environmental Changes/Challenges

As people with DS grow out of the childhood years, changes in the school system, especially when coupled with other stressors, may create enormous strain for them. This strain is often magnified tenfold for teens and young adults with DS-ASD.

The small school and single class of the elementary years gives way to bigger middle schools and high schools and the need to adapt to far larger and more complex settings. These settings have more students and staff and the potential to cause intolerable sensory overstimulation for people with DS-ASD.

Finally, the ability to communicate the cause, source, or presence of a problem is often very difficult for teens and adults with DS, but even more difficult for people with DS-ASD. Many times it seemed that the only recourse people with DS-ASD had to let others know they were stressed was to shut down or to become agitated or aggressive, especially as the stress became more and more intolerable to them.

Compounding of Problems and Issues

We also found a tendency for there to be a compounding of problems and issues. It is fairly easy to see how this happens. There are many possible points of stress or areas of vulnerability for people with DS-ASD, which may include sleep, mystifying hormonal changes, eating problems, bowel and urinary function or dysfunction, more severe communication limitations, a limited number of persons in one's support system (due in part to lack of social skills and relatedness), a tendency toward rigidity in one's daily routine (obsessive compulsive behaviors), and a much higher sensitivity or reaction to sensory stimuli (sensory integration). Add to this the higher incidence of health issues affecting people with DS (hypothyroid, sleep apnea, celiac disease, gastrointestinal issues), and, of course, major environmental changes that are inevitable as children enter middle school and high school years.

Each one of these areas of vulnerability may create a major stressor, but they tend to have a negative effect on other areas as well. In other words, one major change or series of changes can set off a snowball effect, which then results in what families often called a "breakdown" or a "shut down." In these instances, the person with DS-ASD typically shows more extreme forms of behavior, such as aggression toward himself and others, and/or refusal to respond to or cooperate with caregivers around any activity.

Getting Control of the Problem

As mentioned previously, the families in our sample had varying degrees of knowledge about autism when they arrived at our Center. Some were very informed, others were less informed, but we found all were very open to, and interested in, identifying and resolving problems arising from areas of vulnerability and stress. Despite the severity of symptoms and behaviors, and the fact that many families came to us in crisis, we found they had a number of strengths and resources in the family. Many families were also able to find help from our Center and from others in the community, which allowed creative and fruitful ways to get people back on track.

Strengths of the Families in the Sample

Despite, again, the severity of symptoms and behaviors facing these families, especially when there was a crisis or a "breakdown," we found that most of the families had great resilience. Perhaps this is because they had weathered so many different problems and crises over the years. They were weary and even "shell shocked" from the more extreme challenges they encountered for their children in the teen and adult years, but they were still determined to solve these new challenges. We found there were a number of good reasons why they were able to do this. First, most parents and their children with DS-ASD had learned to better communicate, respect, and respond to each other. Parents are quite often very good observers and interpreters to begin with, but most of these parents fine-tuned this skill to understand even subtle cues from their son's or daughter's behavior. This, in turn, had a positive effect on child-parent relationship.

We also found that these families were far more patient and more accepting of their son's and daughter's idiosyncrasies and odd behaviors (e.g., sniffing, staring, hand flapping, mouth noises, etc.). This too helped to reduce the tension and stress between the parent and the teen or adult child. Additionally, even for those who had not been diagnosed previously, the label of autism did not seem to carry the same negative onus as is often experienced by younger families.

Diagnosing ASD in Adults with Down Syndrome

The diagnosis of autism is a deductive process conducted by a group of specialists who are trained in ASD evaluations. After completing a thorough evaluation, the specialists compare the results with the characteristics described in the current edition of the *Diagnostic and Statistical Manual* (DSM) of the American Psychiatric Association or in the *International Classification of Diseases* (IDC) of the World Health Organization, Geneva, Switzerland, both international systems used in the classification of mental disorders. The purpose of the evaluation is to obtain a profile of functioning that will be used for developing appropriate interventions. Early diagnosis of autism is important, as the sooner treatment starts, the better the prognosis, both individually and for the family. Parents who are trained to help their young children with ASD improve their response to the environment report less family stress.

The diagnosis of autism in the general population relies on the use of instruments that assess the presence of behaviors typically associated with ASD. The gold standard of autism assessment is based on an interdisciplinary assessment that includes:

- A complete *medical history,* which should include prenatal and neonatal information, developmental history, family history, medical and educational history, and any prior interventions. A detailed history of sensory issues is also included.

- A complete *medical evaluation* to determine whether there are any physical problems that may account for the behavioral difficulties and to rule out other genetic disorders that could account for the behaviors (e.g., fragile X syndrome, tuberous sclerosis, etc.). It is also important to rule out a significant hearing impairment.
- A *psychological evaluation* to assess cognitive functioning, adaptive behaviors, and the presence of autism.
- A *speech and language evaluation* to assess communicative intent and ability.
- An *occupational therapy evaluation* to assess sensory and motor problems typically associated with autism
- A *psychosocial evaluation* to assess the individual's home and school environment.

The content and diagnostic process will vary depending on the individual's age and history, whether prior evaluations were conducted, and the individual's general level of functioning. Usually the evaluation starts with the family's suspicion that there is something different or problematic with their child's functioning.

The diagnosis of autism in adults with Down syndrome is complicated because of several factors, which include:

- The lack of appropriate diagnostic tools;
- The reliance on caregivers' memory to recall behaviors that existed in early childhood;
- The lack of professional knowledge that both diagnoses may coexist;
- The scarcity of professionals trained to appropriately diagnose autism in adults with Down syndrome.

Despite the above difficulties, the diagnosis of ASD in adults with Down syndrome is possible and should be conducted by professionals experienced in recognizing ASD in individuals with intellectual disabilities. In order to appropriately diagnose ASD in adults with Down syndrome, caregivers need to understand that the diagnosis is a process that cannot be accomplished in one office visit. Unfortunately, there is no blood test that allows us to determine whether an individual has ASD. Perhaps in a few years and as genetic findings continue to advance, this test will become available.

How to Prepare for an ASD Evaluation of an Adult with Down Syndrome

The first step in the diagnostic process is to gather a very detailed medical history. It is important that caregivers provide the diagnostic team with complete medical records, if possible, prior to the first appointment. This gives the team an opportunity to review the records and prepare pertinent questions. We also recommend that the caregivers review both childhood and current pictures and videos to aid in the recollection of early history.

The gold standard for the autism evaluation of teens and adults with Down syndrome is a clinical diagnosis by the multidisciplinary clinical team. Therefore, the teen or adult suspected of having ASD has to be prepared to meet a number of professionals over a period of a few clinic visits. Professionals also have to be sensitive to the difficulties that the person with suspected DS-ASD might have in working with a number of unknown people. Efforts should be made to schedule shorter sessions, be sensitive to sensory issues, and provide many breaks to facilitate the evaluation.

Diagnosing ASD in Teens and Adults with Down Syndrome

The most difficult aspect of the diagnosis of ASD in adults with Down syndrome is identifying appropriate instruments, which would allow the interdisciplinary team to determine the appropriate clinical diagnosis. Expert clinicians are using a number of tools that aid in the diagnosis of ASD in this population. For example, the two gold standard tools for the assessment of ASD are the Autism Diagnostic Interview-Revised (ADI-R) and the Autism Diagnostic Observation Schedule (ADOS).

The ADI-R is a very detailed interview conducted with the parents or caregivers(s). It assesses early and current history of ASD behaviors. The ADOS is an observational tool used for the diagnosis of ASD from toddlers to adults. The ADOS does not provide materials or diagnostic algorithms for nonverbal adolescents and adults with ASD. Thus, when testing a nonverbal adult or teen with Down syndrome and possible ASD, it is important to combine information from all sources, including medical history, history of restricted and repetitive behaviors, creative play, obsessions, stereotyped behaviors, etc.

Activities from the ADOS allow the assessment of current communication and social relationship issues, as well as the observation of behaviors that are typically seen in individuals with ASD (e.g., lack of eye contact, difficulties with reciprocity, etc.). It is important for caregivers to understand that the examiner is observing how the individual behaves with someone he does not know and how he regulates social interaction.

The ADI-R is a very detailed interview with the parents or other caregiver(s) that is used to assess the history and current presence of behaviors also related to ASD. The ADI-R can be used with teens and adults suspected of having ASD, as long as their mental age is above 2 years, 0 months. The interview evaluates three functional domains: 1) language/communication; 2) reciprocal social interaction; 3) restricted, repetitive, and stereotyped behaviors and interests.

The Aberrant Behavior Checklist (Aman & Singh, 1986; Aman, Singh, Stewart & Field, 1995) is also used for assessing problem behaviors in children and adults with intellectual disabilities. The scale provides information in five areas: 1) irritability and agitation; 2) lethargy and social withdrawal; 3) stereotypic behavior; 4) hyperactivity and noncompliance; and 5) inappropriate speech.

Assessing cognitive functioning is important in order to develop the best interventions that are consistent with the individual's functioning. However, cognitive assessment is complicated by the lack of appropriate norms. That is, none of the tests used to assess IQ have been normed, or tested on a large number of people with Down syndrome to determine what the average, below average, and above average range of scores is for each subtest for individuals with DS. Nor have any of the tests been normed on people with DS-ASD. The Leiter-R is a nonverbal cognitive test that is better suited to use with individuals with intellectual disabilities than are the more commonly used tests such as the Wechsler or Stanford-Binet. However, the test requires the understanding and use of gestures, which is difficult for individuals with ASD. One group of researchers suggests the use of a developmental quotient score as a way to calculate how much an individual's skill level deviates from his or her chronological age (De Pellegrino et al., 2010). This method may be used when selecting an assessment tool that was developed for individuals in an age range different from that of the individual being tested (e.g., the Wechsler scales).

The assessment of adaptive behaviors is another area that is helpful when selecting appropriate testing instruments and when creating developmentally appropriate interventions. Understanding what the individual is capable of doing is the foundation to the development of successful strategies to improve lacking skills.

A current speech and language evaluation is helpful to determine the extent of the person's communicative intent and speech and language ability. If possible, this evaluation should be conducted prior to the psychological evaluation. Understanding the person's speech abilities will aid in the selection of the most appropriate cognitive assessment tool, and the appropriate ADOS module.

Individuals with Down syndrome and ASD have sensory and motor problems that may impede normal functioning. An occupational and physical therapy evaluation may therefore aid in determining the most appropriate interventions and/or environmental changes needed.

Finally, an understanding of the individual's current home and school environment is important to facilitate the development of treatment strategies. In addition, a psychosocial assessment by a psychologist, social worker, or a related professional, on the issues discussed at some length in the section on "Current Problems and Issues Identified at the Center" (above), provides clear guidelines as to what services are needed to improve the individual's community functioning.

When conducting an ASD assessment for individuals with Down syndrome, it is important to remember that there are some behaviors that are present in both DS and DS-ASD but that look different when the individual has ASD. For example, obsessional behaviors are present in both DS and DS-ASD, but there are qualitative differences. For example, the compulsions of someone with DS-ASD are more likely to be less functional or out of sync with normal activities or patterns of behavior (e.g., arranging toys in a rigid manner). In contrast, for a person with just DS, the obsessional behavior is more likely to involve the repetition of a more functional behavior (e.g., rigidly adhering to a schedule or routine).

Also keep in mind that difficulties in social relatedness may be due to a hearing impairment or may be part of ASD. Distinguishing ASD behaviors from behaviors associated with the level of cognitive impairment is also a diagnostic challenge. For example, adults with significant levels of intellectual disability may engage in repetitive, stereotyped movements whether or not they have ASD.

Every effort should be made to include a variety of instruments and interviews to aid in the refinement of the ASD diagnosis. The best approach is to consult an interdisciplinary team with experience in diagnosing ASD in adults with Down syndrome.

Differential Diagnosis

When a teen experiences a loss of skill or function, it is important to rule out any other possible causes or explanations other than autism. Ideally, the person can

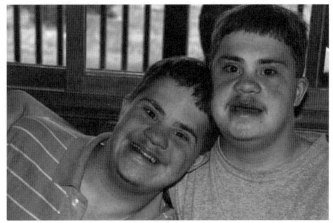

be evaluated at a multidisciplinary clinic staffed by health and mental health professionals who can look at a wide variety of health, sensory (vision and hearing), and environmental stressors that may be associated with a loss of function. When there are symptoms or behaviors of concern, we recommend considering the following:

Communication. People with DS have expressive language limitations and they cannot always communicate the cause or source of problems, even when they have a considerable degree of emotional or physical discomfort or pain. Many times parents and other caregivers are extremely good observers and interpreters of people with DS in their care. We recommend including parents/caregivers in any evaluations to help to better communicate possible issues and concerns for the person with DS.

Lower functioning individuals. Many people who have significant expressive and adaptive skill limitations may appear to have autism because of more extreme communication limitations and stereotypic behaviors. It is important to gather information from knowledgeable informants in the person's residence, work, and recreation settings. The presence or absence of social skills and relatedness is often very easy to discern by credible and caring caregivers who are often excellent interpreters and observers of the individual's subtle and not-so-subtle nonverbal communication.

Social deprivation. Some home and community environments may deprive people of the opportunity to learn social skills and social relatedness. It is not that these individuals cannot learn, just that they have not had adequate training or experience. In most cases, it is possible to tell whether the person has social skills and the ability to learn them by observing how the person acts with other people.

Sensory issues. People with DS have a high incidence of vision and hearing difficulties, which may make them appear unresponsive and unaware of their social and natural environments. Hearing and vision testing is highly recommended. Also, as mentioned previously, many people with DS have sensory processing or sensory integration disorders. A sensory evaluation by an experienced occupational therapist who is trained to evaluate SI problems is highly recommended.

Health issues. People with DS are at greater risk for a number of health issues that may create a significant change in mood or behavior. The most common of these issues include hypothyroidism or hyperthyroidism, sleep apnea, and celiac disease (but there are many others). A complete physical exam by a knowledgeable physician or medical professional is highly recommended to diagnose and treat any health conditions.

Additionally, pain and medical illness may have a significant effect on the person's mood and behavior. It is important to note that many people with DS have a higher threshold of pain. When coupled with communication problems (above), this may delay diagnosis and treatment.

Mental health and behavioral problems. We have seen a number of individuals at the Center who have mental health and behavioral disorders that may generate concern about the possibility of autism. The disorders of greatest concern include depression, trauma, obsessive compulsive disorder (OCD), obsessional slowness, and attention deficit disorder. These disorders will be discussed in more detail later.

First, it is very important to discuss the interaction of mental, physical, sensory, and environmental causes. In our experience, too often people are referred for psychiatric treatment without looking for and treating underlying causes and precipitants, and, as a result, these conditions may continue or worsen. This is particularly the case for a person with DS who cannot easily verbalize or articulate the cause or source of problems. We cannot stress enough the need to look for and treat any and all health and sensory problems as well as to identify and reduce environmental stressors that may be associated with a mental health behavioral problem. We have written extensively about these issues in our writings (McGuire & Chicoine, 2006; Chicoine & McGuire, 2010).

Depression

Depression is one of the most common mental health problems reported for persons with DS (McGuire & Chicoine, 2006; Chicoine & McGuire, 2010). There are a number of reasons for this. First, people with DS are more susceptible to health problems that are a known cause of depression, such as hypothyroid disorder (affecting at least 40 percent of this population), as well as sleep apnea and celiac disease (Chicoine & McGuire, 2010). Second, sensory and sensory processing difficulties are more common, and these too create stress and tend to isolate the individual, placing him more at risk for depression. Many people with DS may also be more susceptible to depression because of expressive language limitations, which may make it more difficult to identify and resolve situations that are stressful to them.

Of the individuals diagnosed with depression at the Adult Down Syndrome Center (McGuire & Chicoine, 2010), those with more severe forms of depression have sometimes seemed to have autistic symptoms to their caregivers. Severe depression often results in a more extreme form of withdrawal. Many people with severe depression refuse to leave the house to go to work or to social events and may stop socializing with family. Many develop odd or unproductive compulsive behaviors, and those who are verbal quite often have agitated self-talk. Perhaps most disturbing to families is the development of a self-absorbed state that takes more and more of the person's attention and focus. Typically, this includes self-talk; even if the person does not talk out loud to himself, he may appear to be communicating with some invisible person or entity. In this state, people appear to be out of touch with the world and reality. Many times parents and other caregivers report that it is often very difficult to pull people back from this self-absorbed state. This is what caregivers can mistake for autism.

With more severe forms of depression, the difference between autism and depression may be difficult to sort out. What we have found is that individuals with more severe depression may stay in a self-absorbed state (described by family members as being "out of it" or "in another world"). This may last for months or years, but still there will be some improvement in time. At first, the individual may show a small but gradually increasing interest in things that he enjoyed previously, such as music, movies, sports, etc. After this, most people gradually return to recreational activities, and then finally they will return to work. Most importantly, with time people regain enough of their social awareness and responsiveness to function adequately in social, recreational, and vocational settings. Some may not return to the level of function they had prior to the onset of their depressed symptoms, but still regain enough skills to relate to others in the different environments they inhabit.

In comparison, a person with DS-ASD who has regressed in social skills and relatedness may be able to go through the motions of relating to others with behavioral training. However, even years later the quality of the social relatedness remains quite deficient.

Trauma

We have seen a number of individuals with Down syndrome who we either know or suspect were severely traumatized by physical or sexual abuse or some other traumatic experience. In response to the trauma, many developed symptoms that are very similar to those described above for individuals with more severe forms of depression. Typically, however, the trauma sufferers also have a considerable amount of anxiety.

Many caregivers suspect trauma when the person with DS avoids activities and places that had been a normal and often an enjoyable part of their daily routine. For example, one woman who was sexually abused at her worksite adamantly refused to go to her job, which was the site of the sexual violence. Many others also have general anxiety and fearfulness, and many are fearful of leaving the home or of going to public places, especially places where there are strangers. Additionally, many people regress and become more dependent on others. They may also become more clingy and afraid to be alone or apart from significant others. Again, what is most disturbing to families is the development of a state of self-absorption very similar to that of individuals who are experiencing more severe forms of depression. The self-absorption often takes more and more of the person's attention and focus. In this state, individuals will appear to be out of touch with the world and reality, and, again, this may look very much like autism.

As with the severely depressed, people with DS who are exposed to a severe trauma may take years to recover, but over time there are significant improvements in social relatedness—which will generally not occur for people with DS-ASD.

Obsessive Compulsive Disorder

As discussed previously, we have found that most people with DS have obsessive compulsive tendencies that we have called "grooves," because people tend to have set patterns and routines in their lives (McGuire & Chicoine, 2006). Under stress, a normally productive groove can become an unproductive obsession or compulsion for many people with DS. We have found that the development of a more rigid or less functional groove is a very common way for people with DS to express stress. If the stress continues, the groove may become an obsession or compulsion that may then begin to interfere in some essential area of life. For example, people may choose to arrange and rearrange personal items or objects in their room rather than to attend a beneficial social or recreational activity that they would normally enjoy.

Obsessions and compulsions may be more odd, extreme, or dysfunctional for teens and adults with DS-ASD compared to those with "just" DS. Still, we have found that many people with DS also have very odd, unusual, and debilitating types of obsessive compulsive disorder (OCD), particularly in response to more extreme stressors in their lives. Therefore, we recommend being very careful in assuming that someone has autism on the basis of obsessions or compulsive behaviors.

Obsessional Slowness

One of the most unusual and frustrating patterns of behavior diagnosed in teens and adults with DS is a condition called obsessional slowness. This condition occurs in a relatively small number of individuals, but for these individuals, the disorder is quite debilitating and it is maddening to caregivers. Sometimes the slowness gradually develops over a period of time, such as months or even years, but other times it may come on suddenly after the person with DS has had a relatively "normal" pattern of behavior for their life.

These individuals move at a pace that is so slow that they cannot go about their daily life and activities without hands-on help and assistance from caregivers. These individuals do not seem to lose the ability to do tasks; rather, their speed prohibits completion in a manner required for life. Additionally, many show very brief bursts of normal speed, but the vast majority of time, movement is painstakingly slow.

Adding greatly to the mystery and frustration of this condition is the fact that no effective treatments have been found to date. In the vast majority of cases, this condition appears to be impervious to psychotropic medications. Some practitioners have found some success with behavioral strategies, but usually even this only provides a small increase in the slow pace.

Because people with obsessional slowness display periods of normal speed, caregivers may wonder if the individual's behavior is purposeful. Caregivers who have observed the slowness over many months and years, however, often come to believe that the individuals who have this conditions have little control over their own pace.

Although parents may be concerned that obsessional slowness is a symptom of autism, most people who have the condition continue to be socially aware and responsive to others. Therefore, caregivers may be dismayed and frustrated by this condition, but the fact that there is a continuation of social relatedness means this is most likely not related to autism.

ADHD

Attention deficit disorder with and without hyperactivity occurs in teens and adults with DS just as it does in the general population. People with DS plus ADHD typically have attention problems, are distractible, and have difficulty controlling their impulses. Individuals with DS-ASD may also be diagnosed with ADHD. The problem for these individuals is not that they are diagnosed with ADHD, but that sometimes they are only given this diagnosis when, in fact, an autism spectrum disorder is present.

Therefore, despite the presence of ADHD symptoms or behaviors, we strongly recommend that a

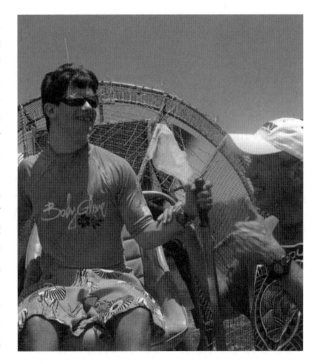

more thorough assessment be made, particularly in terms of social skills and relationship issues, if there are suspicions of possible autism spectrum issues.

ADSC's Role and Interventions That Work

The Adult Down Syndrome Center does not have a diagnostic team for autism. Fortunately, there are several diagnostic centers with whom we can refer and collaborate. Once the diagnosis is made by one of these centers, the person with DS will invariably return to be followed at the ADSC to take advantage of our programs and services.

ADSC staff include a medical team consisting of the third author, one other physician, a nurse practitioner, a nutritionist, three medical assistants, a practice manager, and two administrative staff. Additionally, the psychosocial team includes the first author and two experienced advocacy and outreach staff.

Multidisciplinary Approach. At the ADSC, we take a multidisciplinary approach because we find that problems are often the result of a complex interplay of biological, social, and psychological factors. The multidisciplinary team allows the best means for identifying and treating the different factors at play in a problem. This is especially important for teens and adults with DS-ASD because there are so many areas of vulnerability.

For example, the medical staff identify and treat health problems that occur more frequently in individuals with DS (both with and without ASD). This helps to reduce one very important area of vulnerability. For example, people in this group are just as susceptible to such problems as thyroid disorders, celiac disease, GI problems, and sleep apnea as others with DS.

The psychosocial staff and medical staff also work collaboratively to diagnose and treat mental health and behavioral problems. When deemed appropriate by the team, psychotropic medications may be prescribed to help reduce agitation and get the more disruptive or aggressive behavior under better control. Once agitation is reduced, sleep often improves. Medication can also help to reduce depressive withdrawal, as well as compulsive behavior, which allows people to be more flexible in responding to their world.

Visual Cues. Additionally, once the disruptive behavior is better controlled, we are able to use behavioral strategies more effectively. We have found visual cues to be especially effective in helping teens and adults with DS-ASD learn skills, solve problems, communicate, and manage day-to-day functions and frustrations—regardless of what age the cues are introduced. For example, visual cues can help to make the effects of hormonal changes more understandable and manageable. Visual checklists give women a stepwise means to deal with tasks related to menstruation, and calendars help to show when their periods will occur. For both men and women, sex education charts of the human body help to better show how developmental changes occur in adolescents. Even nocturnal emissions are more understandable to men if they can look at charts of the male reproductive system. It is a little more difficult to use visual supports to explain changes in mood and irritability, but at least the cues give individuals some indication as to why they are having problems.

Visual cues are also very helpful in reducing a common area of stress in the family—completing daily living tasks. Visual cues can help people with DS-ASD to do their tasks without interference or supervision, which gives them a needed sense of control and independence.

Visual cues also give parents "the best shot" at managing eating problems. Most parents are willing to try something new after repeated failures with their attempts to enforce "normal" eating habits. Pictures of the food items and a checklist that are appealing to the individual with DS-ASD can be used. This gives a greater sense of independence and control, as well as a much better chance at a more balanced diet and a calmer meal.

In addition, bowel and bladder issues are better managed with visual cues, helping to reduce another very intense and stressful issue for many families. For example, visual cues can be an effective way to teach basic toileting skills to teens or adults who have not yet mastered them.

We have found that many families have been able to use the most up-to-date technology to incorporate visual cues into their adult child's life. For example, they use smart phones with applications that all teens and adults consider helpful and "cool," instead of the old augmentative devices that are often not used because they were too big and clunky and because they can be embarrassing for teen or young adult users. Smart phones are a far more acceptable way to provide visual cues, and can give people a means to take part in activities they cannot participate in without a visual "checklist" to follow.

Connecting Families with Needed Resources. Our staff also helps families to get in-home behavior management, if they do not already have this service. In-home behavior support is a must for families who are otherwise besieged and overwhelmed by the demands of caring for a son or daughter with DS-ASD. This greatly relieves stress and allows most families to return to some semblance of normalcy.

Our outreach and advocacy staff has also tried very hard to find other appropriate resources and funding sources for sensory evaluations, respite services, and other useful programs and resources for our families. However, despite an obvious need, they often learn that services that are available for children are not always available for teens and adults. Sensory integration evaluations are especially difficult to find, and, when they are available, there are often funding issues. This means that many families have to pay out of pocket for the service, which can be prohibitively expensive.

Critical Need for the Right School or Vocational Program and Staff

For many of the people in our sample, a key precipitant to an eventual "breakdown" was a school or work environment that was not right for them. For most in the sample, one major step to getting things under control was to find a school or work program that was much better suited to their needs. This often included smaller classes, with teachers who were trained and experienced to work with students with ASD or similar types of challenging conditions. Additionally, many families in our sample were able to find special recreation programs staffed by people who were more sensitive to the needs of their son or daughter. This allowed these families peace of mind and a break from the full-time care that had often chained them to their homes.

Family Support

Some of the families in the sample reported that support from extended family and from others in the community became more positive as they accepted the diagnosis. Still, others reported that family and "friends" were not patient or understanding when their son or daughter had an outburst or behaved oddly. They also continued to experience stares and critical looks by others when out of their home and in the community.

On the plus side, many families have found there are far more supports available in the community through local support groups for families with a loved one with DS-ASD and other behavioral challenges. This is due to a combination of things—a greater awareness, over the past ten-plus years, that ASD can co-exist with DS, and of the greater needs of these individuals and their families. For example, in the Chicago area, the National Association for Down Syndrome (NADS) has for the past twelve years run a "parent get-away weekend" for parents with sons and daughters with significant emotional and behavioral challenges (many of whom are diagnosed with ASD). Many of the families in this group look forward to this weekend all year. Ample care is provided for their children with DS-ASD, as well as respite time for their other children. Additionally, the parents hear advice from experts about a host of important topics (behavioral strategies, medication issues, resources, etc.). Perhaps of greatest importance is the support given by the other families at this get-away weekend.

Considering Residence Outside the Home

Like the families of many teens and adults with DS, the families in our sample also considered whether their sons and daughters would benefit from living in a group home. We have discussed these issues at length in the book *The Guide to Good Health for Teens & Adults with Down Syndrome* (Chicoine & McGuire, 2010) and we will not repeat the full discussion here, but a residential option may be especially important to families of a teen or adults with DS-ASD.

We found there were at least two reasons why families in our sample considered group homes. Some looked at group homes when there were no problems occurring at home or in the community. For many, this occurred after a period of crisis and transition into the adult years, but the crisis was dealt with effectively (through in-home and out-of-home behavioral strategies and support, appropriate school or worksites to meet needs, etc). For these families, the residential option was viewed as a natural part of development in the teen and adult years, just as for other sons or daughters who left home.

On the other hand, there were a number of parents whose sons or daughters tended to have more significant challenges and behaviors. These parents considered group homes because they found they could no longer meet their son's or daughter's needs in the teen and adult years. For many, too, the demands of caring for their son or daughter created a major strain on the health and well-being of all family members, including the family member with DS-ASD. Many had also become prisoners in their own homes, not only because of their son's or daughter's behaviors in the community, but also because of the difficulty of finding care-giving help from others.

How did people adapt to the move? Some families were very relieved to find positive changes occurring almost immediately after their son or daughter entered the group home. For others, there was a more tumultuous process of transition. This was very stressful for these families, but it also gave them a glimpse of how competently staff in these homes would deal with behavior in a crisis or transition period. Most of the time, families liked what they saw. Once past the crisis, most individuals with DS-ASD settled in and did very well. The families in both groups have continued to stay very actively involved in their adult children's lives after their moves to group homes.

Summary

People with Down syndrome, with and without ASD, share common characteristics that are often associated with autism. These include repetitious behavior, sensory issues, and communication deficits. Relationship issues appear to be the one area where there is a clear and obvious difference between the two groups. That is, in adults and teens with DS alone, social skills are often a relative strength, whereas in adults and teens with DS-ASD, social skills are a relative weakness.

It is of great importance that professionals who work with teens and adults with Down syndrome familiarize themselves with the behavior characteristics of DS-ASD as well as the medical needs and strategies that are used when ASD is diagnosed in a teen or adult with DS. It is our hope that as the field continues to evolve, ASD will be diagnosed much earlier, since early diagnosis and early intensive interventions allow families to be more successful in managing the ASD characteristics. Autism centers need to be more aware of the coexistence of these two disorders, offer specialized diagnosis, and provide families with the appropriate intervention tools that the field of autism has. An early, multidisciplinary approach to treatment will no doubt benefit the individual with DS-ASD and his or her family.

References

Aman, M. G. & Singh, N. N. (1986). *Aberrant Behavior Checklist: Manual.* East Aurora, NY: Slosson.

Aman, M.G., Singh, N.N., Stewart, A.W., & Field, C.J. (1985). The Aberrant Behavior Checklist. *Psychopharmacology Bulletin.21: 845-50.*

Capone, G. (1999). Down syndrome and autistic spectrum disorder: A look at what we know. *Disability Solutions 3 (5/6):* 8-15.

Chicoine, B. & McGuire, D. (2010). *The Guide to Good Health for Teens & Adults with Down Syndrome.* Bethesda, MD: Woodbine House.

De Pellegrino, G., Fadiga, L., Fogassi, L., Gallese, V., & Rizzolatti, G. (2010). Understanding motor events: A neurophysiological study. *Experimental Brain Research 91:* 176-80.

McGuire, D. & Chicoine, B. (2006). *Mental Wellness in Adults with Down Syndrome: A Guide to Emotional and Behavioral Strengths and Challenges.* Bethesda, MD: Woodbine House.

Medlen, J. (1999). More than Down syndrome: A parent's view. *Disability Solutions 3 (5/6):* 3-7.

Reilly, C. (2009). Autism spectrum disorders in Down syndrome: A review of what we know. *Research in Autism Spectrum Disorders 3:* 829-39.

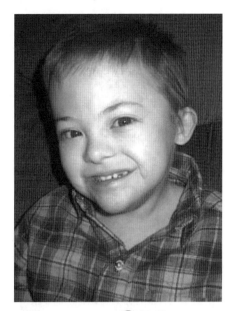

6

Getting the Most Out of Your Doctor Visits

Advice for Parents and Healthcare Providers

Laura Pickler, MD, and Kimberly Bonello

The doctor of the future will give no medicine,
but will interest her or his patients in the care of the human frame,
in a proper diet, and in the cause and prevention of disease.
—Thomas Edison (1847 – 1931)

Before the Visit

Dr. Pickler:
Planning a visit to your child's doctor will be much more productive for everyone involved if you do a little planning prior to making an appointment. If you don't already have a personal physician for your child, a few guiding principles discussed below may be helpful.

Every child deserves a medical home. A medical home is not a specific place or a doctor's office, but conceptually embodies a team approach to health care. These team members include the family, healthcare providers, community programs, insurance, and other payment sources.

According to the American Association of Pediatrics (AAP), there are seven key components to a Medical Home (AAP, 2004):

- Access to care
- Family-centered care
- Cultural responsiveness
- Continuity of care
- Comprehensive care
- Compassionate care
- Coordination of care

One key element in the medical home model of care is the presence of partnerships between the family and all professionals involved in the child's life that together provide a medical home for the child/adult. These partnerships include medical providers but also acknowledge the additional resources that go into quality health care delivery such as school personnel, community therapists, and public health professionals. Also, the rejection of a medical home as a physical location or specific medical practice is important. The patient and family are at the center of the defining statement rather than a specific clinician's office.

Each of the seven components of a medical home becomes linked to some extent to every medical provider of care for the patient with special health care needs as they manage chronic conditions. Familiarity with these components is the first step toward increasing the medical home approach in specialty care. It is completely appropriate for parents to request and expect care to be provided according to the medical home model. Bear in mind, however, that this may look different for each individual family. Parents should feel empowered and encouraged to discuss what this means for their child with their child's primary care provider.

Once you have an established medical home, the following practical suggestions will be easier to implement:

- Make appointments that do not interfere with other activities such as school or therapy sessions if at all possible.
- Consider whether it is better for your family to have multiple appointments in one day to minimize travel, or to only have one appointment in a day to minimize stress.
- Make a list of things you want to discuss. Keep in mind that if your list is long or the items are complex, you may not get every item addressed in one visit.
- Ask for extra time during an appointment when you schedule. If it is difficult to schedule extra time, consider requesting the last appointment of the day so that your doctor isn't rushed. Making sure that your doctor has enough time scheduled to meet your needs will limit the possibility of being kept waiting at the doctor's office.

- Be on time. No one likes to be kept waiting. If you are late, chances are that every family after you will also be seen late. Timeliness is considerate, not just to the doctor and his/her staff, but to every patient scheduled that day after you. Many offices are enacting policies that may ask you to reschedule if you are more than ten minutes late.

If your child is agitated while you wait for your appointment to begin, let a nurse know. There are likely options for limiting or eliminating waiting time at the doctor's office. The practice may also have options for making wait time more pleasant for everyone.

Kim Bonello:

As the mother of a young adult with DS-ASD, I have learned so much from my beautiful daughter, Emily, about how to be a good medical advocate for her as well as for myself and our entire family. I have made many mistakes over the years, and I've learned the hard way how to help streamline and coordinate Emily's medical care. I hope you will benefit from my experiences and decide which of my suggestions you will use on your family's journey with DS-ASD.

It might be helpful to remember that doctors and other healthcare providers are there to serve you and your child. A good doctor will not be offended if you request a second opinion. If it is not working well with a particular provider, please know that you are within your rights to seek a new provider. Being with the wrong doctor/provider will only cause you and your child undue anxiety, while finding the right doctor/provider will ease your mind and empower you to ask the questions you need to ask in order to ensure your child's long-term health and happiness.

With that said, I'd like to offer some suggestions to hopefully make your child's next appointment a little less stressful for both of you:

- Provide as much information as possible to the scheduler about what you want to accomplish during your child's doctor visit so the doctor can be better prepared to address issues of concern.
- When visiting a new doctor or facility, ask the scheduler about location, parking, where to enter the building, and the check-in process so you can be prepared. Ask if they have a website where you can get all that information, as well as any needed forms you can fill out in advance. This will reduce stress on you and your child.
- Tell the scheduler about any special accommodations your child may need, such as wheelchair access, special or more private waiting areas, or immediate room placement to avoid over-stimulation.
- To the extent that your child can understand, tell her about the appointment in advance, such as who will see her and why. For example, I tell Emily, "We are going to see Dr. Pickler [tomorrow, today, in a few minutes]. She will listen to your chest and back and will look in your ears and mouth." Whether there is a response or not, repeat this a few times before the appointment so there are no, or only a few, surprises.

■ Prepare a *"medical resume."* Every doctor, nurse, anesthesiologist, etc. who has received Emily's resume has said, "I wish every parent would prepare one of these!" Keep a copy of your child's resume on your computer or flash-drive so you can update it and print it quickly for appointments. What should you include in your child's medical resume?

- ■ 1st Page: List child's name, address, name of parent/guardian, phone number, insurance information, diagnoses, special notes.
- ■ 2nd Page: List current medications and allergies.
- ■ 3rd Page: List all doctors with addresses, phone and fax numbers, and their specialty (PCP, ENT, Dentist, etc.).
- ■ 4th Page: List studies and tests previously done (CT scans, MRIs, sleep studies, etc.) and their results.
- ■ 5th Page: List all surgeries and/or hospitalizations, including date, facility/hospital, name of doctor, procedure done, and results.

Creating a medical resume will help with the constant requests to explain your child's medical issues. It will also help when filling out forms, as you can write, "see attached medical resume" instead of filling out multiple forms. In order to protect your child's identity, do *not* put her Social Security number on this document.

During the Visit

Dr. Pickler:

Once you have decided when and where your child will be seen, you have completed a great deal of work that will make the actual visit go well. Thinking through the logistics of the initial portion of the appointment is your next step. If your child has sensory sensitivities, bring any items from home that will make it easier if you have to wait to be seen that day. Examples may include snacks, a favorite toy, or a blanket. You might request to be put into a room right away so that your child is away from the noise and activity of the waiting area. Some children enjoy motor activities such as stringing beads, stacking blocks, or coloring while they wait. Whatever you decide will help your child be relaxed and comfortable during the initial process of checking in and waiting to be seen will greatly help when the doctor is in the room discussing your concerns.

Never underestimate the importance of a list. Grocery lists are important for efficiency when you are shopping and so are lists for your medical provider. If possible, prioritize the items you wish to discuss to avoid bringing up your most important concern when the doctor is thinking the visit is almost over. If you make a list, your doctor can know what things are most important to you. Keep in mind that the doctor may not have the same list that you do. He/she may not have prioritized items in the same order that you did. These differences are OK and to be expected. The key to good communication during the visit is to be clear about your needs. Do not be a slave to the list! If items are complex or if your child is sick, you may not get through every item on your list. Some families save their lists from visit to visit to ensure that nothing is forgotten.

Note that there are several types of appointments that may dictate the expectations for how things will progress for the doctor and his/her staff as well as for you and your child. If you are bringing in your child due to an illness or other specific complaint, keep your list brief. Try to focus on the reason for the visit so that adequate time and energy can be spent getting your child the help she needs. I highly recommend also scheduling visits at least every six months when your child is not ill or having an acute problem. This allows for time to receive information about the resources you need to successfully parent your child and to prevent things that may cause problems later. It also makes time for care coordination between the various providers with whom your child has interactions. More frequent visits help keep everyone up to date and provide opportunities to review items on your child's care plan. Most children and adults have a better experience during medical visits if there is a routine in place that is not forgotten between visits.

Kim Bonello:

Your child will learn from each doctor visit and it will get easier in time. Make simple accommodations in order to put your child at ease and lessen her anxiety. This may include turning off florescent lights, removing "crinkly" paper from the exam table, and closing the door if another child is fussing or crying. Bring quiet activities that you have saved just for the doctor visit. Perhaps you can read a favorite book or bring a new coloring book and crayons to enjoy while you're waiting for the doctor to arrive.

Pay attention to your child's cues during the doctor's visit. If something is causing distress, be quick to react in order to head off a meltdown. Tell the doctor what works best for your child. Perhaps you might say, "Be swift about the exam and keep talking softly about what you are doing, but don't ask if you may look in her ears—just do it." Or you may say, "You need to warn her in advance about everything you are going to do and take your time and wait until she's ready to comply." It all depends on what your child needs, and you are the best expert on your child. Help the doctor out by telling him or her what works and what doesn't work. Also, if possible, you may want to request that anything really uncomfortable or painful such as shots be done towards the end of the visit.

Know when it's time to end the visit, even if you haven't accomplished everything or asked every question you had written down. If you need to end the visit abruptly, make an appointment for a follow-up phone call or ask if you can send the doctor an email so you can finish asking your questions. Get as much of the physical exam done as quickly as possible just in case your child reaches her threshold for this visit and needs to leave. If you leave *before* a meltdown occurs, your child will learn to trust that future visits will be tolerable and that you care about her comfort.

When it comes to working with your child's doctor, be helpful and pleasant while he or she is examining your child. You catch more flies with honey than vinegar! If you need to become assertive to get your point across or to get what your child needs, absolutely be assertive. Remember, however, that your goal is to be assertive, not aggressive. Being aggressive will not serve your child in the slightest, but being positively assertive will pay off in a big way.

After the Visit

Dr. Pickler:

At the close of every visit, the parent and provider should both have an understanding of what needs to be done, who will do it, and in what timeframe it will be completed. It is sometimes helpful to make a list so that everyone knows their role. A

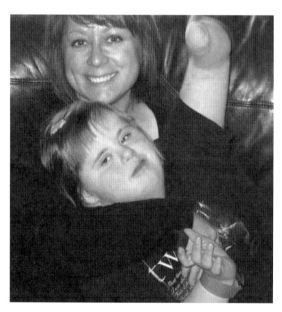

follow-up plan should be decided upon. This can be done either in person or by phone or email. Increasingly, technology is allowing families to manage aspects of their child's care electronically such as by checking lab results or drafting written care plans.

If your practice does not already have a mechanism in place to communicate with a team member who has the role of case manager, explore with the practice whether they can assign this role to someone. This will greatly help with in-person communication between visits and help your family get your needs for paperwork or equipment authorizations met.

Occasionally, a family may desire to play a larger role in their child's medical home than is outlined above. For example, the family may want to organize quality improvement activities in the practice to help with making the practice more family centered, assist other families in connecting with resources or community services, or provide support to other families who also have children with special needs. Most physicians who are committed to providing care in the medical home model will appreciate your efforts and find ways to encourage and support you.

Kim Bonello:

I always offer Emily a reward after she has visited the doctor. Sometimes I use a food reward, because there is a gelato stand in the lobby of her doctor's office and Emily loves gelato. But I also use other rewards, such as a promise to go home and watch a favorite movie and eat popcorn together, a new "stim" toy that she can add to her collection, or letting Emily decide what reward she would like that day. Rewards don't have to cost you anything. A "high five" or a heartfelt "Thank you, Emily" can mean so much to her. She associates going to the doctor with a safe and rewarding experience at this point in her life, and this is what I call a major success!!

A Special Note about Organizing General Anesthesia

Dr. Pickler:

A certain subset of patients with DS-ASD are greatly served by planning to have needed services or procedures that would otherwise be very distressing or significantly uncomfortable performed under anesthesia. A discussion with your doctor about organizing care in this way is important. Risks and benefits to general anesthesia should be carefully considered. Examples of procedures to be considered are below:

- Dental work, deep cleanings, and x-rays
- Any blood monitoring (thyroid panels, medication monitoring labs, etc.)
- Eye health screenings
- Hearing screenings
- Immunization administration
- Gynecological exams
- X-rays, ultrasounds, MRIs, CT scans

Kim Bonello:

Annually, Emily's doctor and I schedule one day to take care of all invasive and challenging procedures that are needed for the entire year. While it takes quite a bit of effort to coordinate the schedules of the dentist, ENT surgeon, radiology/lab, and other specialists, it is well worth it!

In preparation for procedures under anesthesia, discuss with your child's surgical team options for pre-surgery medications that may help ease the anxiety of the entire experience. Perhaps your child would benefit from having a medication such as Versed, which not only relaxes but causes an "amnesia affect," so she will not even remember being brought back to the operating room. If your child will not willingly swallow a pre-surgery medication, ask for alternative methods of delivery, such as injection or a spray into the nasal passages. Pre-surgery medications have worked wonders for Emily and have saved me from watching her have panic attacks or become combative prior to surgery. I always ask the surgical team to have Emily go "under" with the mask *prior* to placing the IV. Emily does not cooperate with having an IV placed while awake, and this way she is unaware of its placement because she is already asleep.

Bear in mind that it can be difficult to get insurance companies to pay for anesthesia for procedures that are not usually done under anesthesia. In my experience, most insurance companies want you to try to do the procedure or appointment in the conventional way. If it is impossible to complete the procedure or exam any other way, then they will pay for anesthesia.

Life is so much easier now that her medical care is more streamlined. Emily's anxiety is diminished, as well as mine. Because we have chosen to have multiple procedures done under anesthesia once a year, Emily is no longer afraid of going to the doctor. It has all become very routine and she knows what to expect. All my best to you as you find the right medical providers who will work with you and help you coordinate a care plan that works well for your entire family.

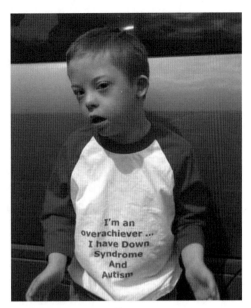

7

What Autism Looks Like in a Child with Down Syndrome
The Behavioral Phenotype

Susan Hepburn, PhD, and Deborah J. Fidler, PhD

Introduction

For years, most professionals and parents regarded the co-occurrence of autism and Down syndrome to be very rare. In fact, given the social strengths that were often reported in children with Down syndrome, it seemed particularly improbable that a condition that impacts social-communication would be evident in a child with Down syndrome.

However, as more and more parents expressed concerns about the different developmental path their sons or daughters with Down syndrome seemed to be taking, clinical researchers began to take note of the possibility that some children with Down syndrome could also be challenged by an additional behavioral diagnosis—an autism spectrum disorder (ASD).

In making a diagnosis of an ASD, a clinician—usually a pediatrician, clinical psychologist, psychiatrist, or neurologist—relies upon the criteria for an ASD that are provided by the most current edition of the *Diagnostic and Statistical Manual of Mental Disorders* (American Psychiatric Association, 2000), which is the medical "guidebook" for diagnoses. These criteria have been fairly stable since they were first developed almost fifty years ago, at least in spirit, although they are under revision again for updating in 2015.

In order for a person to receive a diagnosis of an ASD, he or she must show significant difficulties in three areas of development: 1) social functioning, 2) nonverbal and verbal communication, and 3) restricted interests and activities. Within each of these areas, there are four behavioral indicators, or symptoms, that characterize the type of impairment that is relevant to an ASD.

Within the current diagnostic system (DSM-IV-TR), a diagnosis of Autistic Disorder can be made if there is evidence for at least two or more symptoms in each area; if these symptoms were evident before the child was three years old; if they cause impairment in functioning; and if they can't be explained better by another condition. A diagnosis of Pervasive Developmental Disorder Not Otherwise Specified (PDD-NOS) is made if the clinician finds evidence for some impairment in each of the three areas, but not enough to meet criteria for Autism Spectrum Disorder. Although it may be tempting to assume that a diagnosis of PDD-NOS suggests the child is more mildly affected by autism than a child with the full diagnosis, that assumption is not always true. Some children with PDD-NOS, while showing fewer symptoms, actually demonstrate more severity and impairment in the few symptoms they do have, thus experiencing a more clinically significant version of the condition than a child with a more mild form of more symptoms. In other words, the sheer number of symptoms that are evident is not, in itself, the best way to think about the severity of a child's impairment. Note also that the next revision of the DSM may not include the diagnosis of PDD-NOS at all, but only the single diagnosis of Autism Spectrum Disorder.

Basic Facts about Autism Spectrum Disorders

There are a few other things to know about autism spectrum disorders before we discuss what an ASD can look like in a child with Down syndrome.

1. ASD is a developmental disability that can be identified only through a developmental/behavioral evaluation process. There is no medical test for autism, so the skill and experience of the people evaluating a child with another known developmental disability is especially important in determining if this second condition is in the picture.

2. ASD is a biologically-based condition that involves disorders of development of the nervous system, including the brain.

3. Many different biological systems may or may not be involved in a particular child's ASD; such as the motor system, speech-language system, immune system, sleep/regulatory systems, gastrointestinal system, sensory processing systems (including vision, hearing, tactile sensitivity, taste/smell, vestibular, and pain sensitivity). Researchers are studying the "multi-system" nature of ASD very actively. For updated information on the medical aspects of ASD, check the websites for the American Academy of Pediatrics (www.aap.org/healthtopics/autism.cfm) or the Centers for Disease Control and Prevention (www.cdc.gov/ncbddd/autism).

4. ASD is not caused by poor parenting. Although we do not know the specific causes of ASD, scientists think that the condition is strongly genetic, but in a very complex way, such that several different genetic differences need to happen at the same time in order for the "scene to be set" for an ASD to develop. Then, most scientists think, this "genetic vulnerability" to an ASD needs to be "turned on" by some kind of environmental or experiential factor. This would explain how studies of identical twins (children who share the exact same genetic makeup) report that it is possible for one twin to have an ASD and the other to be developing typically. Or, as happens more often, how one twin can be more severely affected by ASD symptoms than his or her co-twin. Scientists are actively studying the genetics of ASD, and the observation that children with Down syndrome are at particular risk for an ASD is leading some to examine chromosome 21 as a potential site for genes that are relevant to ASD as well. (See Chapter Three.)

5. The biological underpinnings of ASD have not been found to exist in any one part of the brain. Rather, they are more likely to involve problems in the brain's connectivity, or the efficiency with which the brain can send messages across neural structures and integrate information from different brain regions.

6. Recent research suggests that there is an increase in children with ASD throughout the developing world that cannot be accounted for by better diagnostic methods or changes in clinical practice. Current studies suggest that 1 in 91 children has an ASD, which is significantly higher than estimates generated 20 years ago of 1 in 2500 children (Fombonne, 2005). This dramatic increase is being actively studied by epidemiologists, who are examining several environmental and biological factors that may be involved in the increased numbers of children affected worldwide.

7. ASD is reported to occur in children of all different racial, ethnic, and socioeconomic groups. However, there is some evidence for disparities in the age of diagnosis, such that children with higher socioeconomic status, those living near medical centers, and possibly of Caucasian ethnicity tend to receive the diagnosis earlier.

8. ASD is found to occur more often in males; approximately 3 boys are identified for every girl. The reasons for this are unknown, leading researchers to examine x-linked genetic conditions, hormonal influences, and the evolutionary biology of brain development. (For example: Are there differences in the male and female brains? If so, do these differences yield clues to the possible brain regions involved in ASD?)

9. There are a lot of ways that children with a diagnosis of an ASD differ from each other. Clinicians and researchers would say that the disorder is "heterogeneous" or "has a lot of variability." Possible sources of these individual differences in how an ASD presents in each individual child are listed in Table 7-1 on the next page.

Table 7-1 Possible Sources of Individual Differences in Symptom Presentation in ASD

	How Differences Impact Symptom Presentation
Chronological age	Younger children show different forms of social, communicative, and behavioral differences than older children. For example, children with ASD under the age of 3 years rarely understand what simple gestures, such as pointing, mean, and they are not likely to follow an adult's pointed finger with their eye gaze to see what is of interest. However, most kids with ASD learn to follow another person's point by the time they enter kindergarten. Therefore, failure to follow a point is an important symptom to look for in toddlers and preschoolers, but doesn't differentiate children with ASD from others in the school years.
Overall developmental level	A child's overall developmental level is very important to consider when setting expectations for social and communicative skills.
Patterns of cognitive strengths and weaknesses	Some children with ASD are better at solving problems without language, others are better at verbal reasoning. Some children with ASD learn best with lots of visual supports, while others tend to learn better through auditory (e.g., listening) or kinesthetic means (e.g., moving/doing).
Temperament	Behavioral style, one's individual manner of operating in the world, a constitutional tendency to respond to certain situations in predictable ways.
Activity Level	Some children with ASD are highly active and in constant motion. Others are more lethargic, slow to respond, and seem to have difficulty getting started.
Emotional intensity	Some children are very emotionally reactive and show strong feelings regularly. Others may seem unusually nonreactive to emotional or charged situations and experiences.
Adaptability or "behavioral flexibility"	Some children can "go with the flow" better than others and tend to be able to adjust to changes in situations or expectations. Others have intense difficulty being flexible, managing transitions, and integrating new experiences.
Persistence or "mastery motivation"	Some children show a drive to complete a task or achieve a goal of some kind that is remarkably focused. Others give up much more easily, or avoid trying new challenges completely. Many parents report that their children with ASD show different levels of persistence in different tasks/activities (e.g., persistent with a special interest—such as lining up cars—but not persistent in learning to write letters).
Distractibility	Some children are difficult to distract from what they are doing ("overly focused") and others seem distracted ("unfocused") much of the time. And some children show both attentional styles at different times.

10. A diagnosis of ASD is only relevant if a person's difficulties in social functioning and nonverbal communication abilities are more severe than would be expected for the person's developmental level, not his chronological age. For example, let's say that an 8-year-old boy with Down syndrome is functioning more like a 4-year-old. (Note: This kind of developmental estimate can be obtained through standardized testing, accompanied by some assessment of the child's skills and abilities in real life, known as "adaptive functioning," which is usually assessed by interviewing parents and caregivers who know the child well, using a standardized tool such as the Vineland Scales of Adaptive Behavior) (Sparrow, Cicchetti, & Balla, 2005). In this case, the child's chronological age is 8 years and his developmental age is 4 years. If, during a specific evaluation of social reciprocity and nonverbal communication (which are the hallmarks of ASD), the child demonstrates social and nonverbal communicative behaviors that are similar to those seen in a 4-year-old with Down syndrome, then his challenges are interpreted to be part of his developmental delay, but not indicative of a co-occurring ASD. If, however, the child lacks the social and nonverbal communication behaviors seen in most 4-year-olds, then an ASD may be relevant for this child. See Table 7-2 below for an overview of the developmental ages associated with several important social-communication behaviors.

Table 7-2 Developmental Ages Associated with Specific Social-Communicative Behaviors

Social/Communicative Behaviors	Expected age of accomplishment
Expresses a variety of emotions (including happiness, sadness, interest, surprise, anger, fear, disgust)	By the age of 6 months
Demonstrates a predictable social smile (i.e., a smile that is clearly directed at or shared with another person)	By the age of 6 months
Matches the emotions expressed by an adult in face-to-face interactions	By the age of 6 months
Shows nervousness with strangers (and therefore is differentiating familiar and unfamiliar people)	Between 7 and 12 months
Relies on caregiver to be a secure base while exploring environment	Between 7 and 12 months
Uses social referencing (looking back at caregiver) in order to pick up cues about how to react in new situations	Between 7 and 12 months

(continued on next page)

(continued from previous page)

Readily joins in play with familiar children, such as siblings, cousins, etc.	Between 13 and 18 months
Recognizes image of self in mirrors and pictures	Between 13 and 18 months
Begins to show empathy for others (by trying to comfort others or directing sympathetic facial expressions to others who are hurt or unhappy)	Between 13 and 18 months
Able to follow simple directions given by familiar caregiver	Between 13 and 18 months

Social Behaviors	Expected age of accomplishment
Expresses more subtle, more complex emotions, such as shame and embarrassment (these emotions are indicative of developmental growth in social cognition)	Between 19 and 24 months
Verbally expresses a variety of emotion words	Between 19 and 24 months
Begins to use communication as a tool for self-regulation (uses verbal and nonverbal communication to express feelings, make requests)	Between 19 and 24 months
Uses own name and personal pronouns	Between 19 and 24 months
Understands basic categories that are associated with people, such as age and sex	Between 19 and 24 months
Distinguishes between intentional and unintentional acts by self and others	Between 2 and 3 years (25-36 months)
Shows ability to be cooperative with caregivers	Between 2 and 3 years (25-36 months)
Shows emerging understanding of how actions cause feelings and vice versa	Between 2 and 3 years (25-36 months)
Demonstrates greater capacity for empathy, characterized by sharing and increased acts of generosity to comfort others	Between 2 and 3 years (25-36 months)
Expression of complex emotions (such as shame, embarrassment, guilt, pride) increases	Between 3 and 5 years (25-60 months)
Engages in first friendships	Between 3 and 5 years (25-60 months)

Adapted from Berk, L.E. (2009). *Infants, children, and adolescents.* 3rd ed. Boston: Allyn & Bacon

Basic Facts about Down Syndrome

Before we can talk about what autism looks like in a person with Down syndrome, we have to first consider a few points about general development in Down syndrome, when an ASD is not thought to be part of a child's clinical presentation.

1. The incidence rate of Down syndrome is approximately 1 in 691 when averaged across all maternal ages (CDC, 2009). The likelihood of having a child with Down syndrome increases with maternal age, and by age 40, the likelihood of having a child with Down syndrome is approximately 1 in 25.

2. The majority of cases of Down syndrome are caused by "nondisjunction," or a failure in cell division during the formation of gametes (ovum for women, sperm for men). As a result of this failure, when fertilization takes place, three copies of chromosome 21 are found in the fertilized egg instead of two. In other, less frequent cases, cell division errors happen after fertilization, which can lead to "mosaicism." Another rare cause of Down syndrome occurs when a parent passes along a chromosome that has additional information from chromosome 21 attached to it, which is called a "translocation."

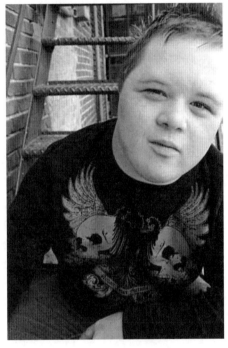

3. Down syndrome affects activity of over 300 genes and their associated proteins and enzymes, and therefore affects multiple systems (Gardiner & Costa, 2006).

4. Down syndrome is associated with specific physical features, including a distinctive craniofacial structure, brachycephaly (abnormally wide head shape), short neck, congenital heart defects, muscular hypotonia, and musculoskeletal hyperflexibility. A unique craniofacial appearance is also found in Down syndrome, which often includes some or all of these features: upslanting palpebral fissures, epicanthal folds, Brushfield spots, flat nasal bridge, dysplastic ear, and a high arched palate.

5. In addition to specific physical features, Down syndrome predisposes an individual to specific behavioral outcomes. Recent work in this area suggests that many individuals with Down syndrome show areas of

relative strength in visual processing, language understanding, and some aspects of social relatedness. Challenges have been reported in the areas of expressive language, auditory processing, and some aspects of movement development. It is important to note that not every individual with Down syndrome will show all aspects of the behavioral profile. Rather, the likelihood that individuals with Down syndrome will show this pattern of outcomes is higher than in other children with developmental disabilities who do not have Down syndrome.

6. The majority of children with Down syndrome score in the mild (55-70) to moderate (40-55) range of cognitive impairment, though the range of outcomes includes mild to profound impairments. Over the first few years of life, most children with Down syndrome make steady progress in development, but they do not make these gains at the same rate as other children without disabilities. Thus, their IQ scores tend to become gradually lower throughout childhood.

7. Speech and expressive language skills tend to be delayed in Down syndrome relative to nonverbal abilities. However, receptive language (language understanding) seems to develop with relative competence in Down syndrome, with the majority of children aged birth to five showing mental-age appropriate receptive language skills. While the majority, but not all, children with Down syndrome show a profile of relative strengths in receptive over expressive language, there may be different pathways leading to this outcome.

8. Many children with Down syndrome generally show delays in the transition from prelinguistic communication to meaningful speech. Young children with Down syndrome may show an average productive (signed or spoken) vocabulary of 28 words at 24 months, 116 words at 36 months, 248 words at 48 months, and 330 words at 72 months. When considering only spoken (not signed) vocabulary words, only 12 percent of one-year-olds with Down syndrome have produced their first words, and only 53 percent of four-year-old children have vocabularies larger than 50 words, a level that would be on par with a typically developing 16-month-old child.

9. The use of gestures in children with Down syndrome seems to be an area of strength, and some studies report that individuals with Down syndrome use more advanced gestures than expected based on their general language development levels, and a wider repertoire of functional, symbolic, and pretending gestures than typically developing children at the same language level.

10. Young children with Down syndrome show mental age-appropriate levels of nonverbal joint attention, or the use of eye contact, gesture, and vocalization for the purposes of social sharing, according to most studies. But difficulties are observed in nonverbal requesting behav-

iors, or the use of eye contact, gesture, or vocalization for the purposes of obtaining a certain outcome (a desired toy, food item, etc).

11. Motor development is an area of delay in many children with Down syndrome. Atypical development of reflexes, low muscle tone, and hyperflexibility are often observed.

12. During early development, many children with Down syndrome reach social relatedness milestones with competence. Infants with Down syndrome show longer looking times at people versus objects, and show increased melodic sounds, vocalic sounds, and emotional sounds when interacting with people rather than objects (Legerstee, Bowman, & Fels, 1992). Toddlers with Down syndrome also achieve competence in the areas of joint attention, sharing objects with others, and other social initiations. Socialization skills in the school years have often been cited as an area of strength within the larger area of adaptation.

13. Many individuals with Down syndrome may show difficulty with aspects of problem solving and goal-directed behavior. Some individuals may develop a style in which they abandon difficult tasks more quickly than other children.

14. Individuals with Down syndrome may have some difficulty with perspective taking and understanding other people's motives, desires, and feelings.

15. Down syndrome may predispose some children to specific behavior problems, including oppositionality, inattentiveness, and hyperactivity. Other conditions, such as anxiety and depression, are reported to occur less frequently in children with Down syndrome than in other children with developmental disabilities, but their rates are higher than in typically developing children. Issues related to mood may become more common during transitions to adolescence and as individuals reach adulthood.

ASD in Children with Down Syndrome: A Different Clinical Presentation?

As noted in Table 7-2, one of the important sources of individual differences in how an ASD presents is whether or not the child has another diagnosis that affects behavior or development. This brings us to the mission of this chapter, which is to describe how an ASD is likely to present in a child with Down syndrome—which, we believe (as do others in the field), has a characteristic "feel" or clinical picture. That is, while children with both Down syndrome and ASD have many things in common, there is a particular "flavor" to the condition when a child has both conditions. In our clinical experience, the presentation is unique—different from what we see in children with Down syndrome alone or ASD alone.

In other words, having both conditions (Down syndrome + ASD) may be a qualitatively different experience from having either one alone—both for the child and for the family. In the sections that follow, we will try to share our clinical observations about how the co-occurrence impacts the child. Family issues will be discussed elsewhere in this volume.

The Behavioral Phenotype of Down Syndrome and ASD

We thought we'd try to use a case study approach to illustrate how having an ASD might impact the behavior of a person with Down syndrome. In order for this approach to make sense, we need to think developmentally. Therefore, we will describe four children with Down syndrome and ASD, of differing developmental levels and ages, whom we have had the chance to get to know very well through various research studies. We will also describe four of their peers with Down syndrome alone, who are similar in both chronological and mental age as the child with both Down syndrome and ASD. As with any case study approach, we want to emphasize that these examples do not provide a comprehensive view of how the two disorders can co-occur. As discussed previously, there is a multitude of ways that an ASD can present in any person, but hopefully these case examples will serve to show some of the more common patterns we tend to observe. In order to protect confidentiality, we are changing names and other details not germane to the contrast we are trying to illustrate.

Preschool-Aged Children

Preschool-Aged Children who Currently Function More Like 12- to 18-month-olds
- Chronological Age: 3½ years (42 months)
- Developmental Age: 12-16 months

Wade: Child with Down Syndrome without ASD. Wade is a sweet, quiet boy with very low muscle tone and difficulty coordinating his body. He scoots his body on the floor in a sort of "commando crawl" and is working on walking. He laughs and smiles when his parents or therapists talk to him and praise his efforts at using his body. He loves music and watches his mother's face intently when she sings to him. If she pauses in the middle of a line in a song that he knows well, he moves his hand excitedly, makes a sound, and looks at his mom with a smile. When she continues the song, he giggles and pats her face. When his mom claps at the end of a song, he tries to do the same but his hand control makes it hard to clap effectively. This doesn't appear to frustrate him and he smiles gleefully. Wade likes to play pat-a-cake and tries to do the movements his mom shows him. When she hugs him, he cuddles his body into her. When she calls his name, it takes him a few seconds to turn his head, but he usually turns toward the sound of her voice. Wade vocalizes often while looking at another person, but is not yet using words. His favorite activities are cause-and-effect musical toys, singing songs with his mom, and playing in water or sand. He loves the family dog and playing near his big sister.

Ryan: Child with Down Syndrome and ASD. Ryan is a quiet, endearing little boy who looks sort of serious much of the time. He has low muscle tone, and learned to walk when he was about two years old. Ryan doesn't seem to like being praised by his parents or therapists and sometimes he covers his ears when they clap for him. He likes music, especially when it is sung softly. Ryan will back his body into his mother's and pull her hands around him, moving her body almost as if he is adjusting a piece of furniture to sit on. His mom is very good at knowing what he wants and she sings one of his two favorite songs when he does this. During the singing, he rocks in her lap, looking forward. When she pauses the song, he becomes distressed and cries, pulls at her body without looking at her, and then gets up and walks away. He doesn't seem to know how to let her know that he would like to hear more. Ryan's mom tries to engage him in pat-a-cake and peek-a-boo, but he walks away. When Ryan is really happy, he laughs and jumps up and down and vocalizes gleefully, but he doesn't look at others or do things to share his emotion. When his mother calls his name, he rarely looks up or pays attention—in fact, his parents wondered if he was deaf and sought hearing tests to rule out a hearing impairment. He isn't yet imitating sounds or gestures, like waving goodbye. His favorite activities are playing with string, swinging, and water play. When his older sister tries to get him to play, he seems to ignore her or walks away.

WHAT TO NOTICE

In these two examples, we have a preschool-aged child who is functioning more like a 12- to 16-month-old, so we want to think about the social and communication skills we would hope to see in a typically developing child at that age. If the child has most of these skills, then an ASD is probably not present. In the example above, Wade has many of the social-communication skills we would expect in a 12- to 16-month-old. These are discussed below.

Sharing Affect: Young children direct their facial expressions toward others to share their feelings.

WHAT DOES WADE DO: When happy, Wade smiles and directs this smile to his mom in order to share the experience. When sad or frustrated, we expect that Wade probably directs his face toward his caregiver to share that feeling as well.

WHAT DOES RYAN DO: When happy, Ryan doesn't tend to look at others and share a smile, nor does he direct his distress or frustration toward others. He experiences emotions, sometimes quite strongly, but he doesn't recruit others into his experience or seem to try to share how he is feeling.

Shows a Range of Affect: Young children's feelings change frequently and fluidly, depending upon what is happening around or within them. Caregivers can usually tell how they are feeling from their affect—their facial expressions, bodily postures, and the quality of their vocalizations.

WHAT DOES WADE DO: Even with his motor challenges, Wade uses his face, eyes, and body to send messages about how he is feeling that his mom can understand most of the time. His emotions seem to make sense, given what is happening around him.

WHAT DOES RYAN DO: Ryan has a somewhat flat, or less variable, facial expression much of the time. It can be hard to know how he is feeling. His emotions seem hard to predict and he can become intensely upset, even though it doesn't seem like anything is happening to cause the distress. Sometimes he laughs when others cry.

Sharing Attention with Another Person: Young children learn about the world by focusing on the same activity as another person and thus building skills, such as word learning, by being "on the same page" as a caregiver.

WHAT DOES WADE DO: During the song games with his mom, Wade participates with her, clearly sharing attention on the song. If his mom showed him a book, Wade would look at the pictures she was showing him.

WHAT DOES RYAN DO: During the song game with his mom, Ryan doesn't participate actively and abandons the shared activity early. If his mom showed him a book, it is likely that Ryan would not look at the book with her, even briefly.

Responding to His Name: Young children with good hearing and motor control will turn their heads toward their caregiver's voice when their name is called. This is an early emerging form of social orienting.

WHAT DOES WADE DO: Even with his motor challenges, Wade attempts to turn his head toward the sound of his mother's voice and it is clear that he knows she wants his attention.

WHAT DOES RYAN DO: Ryan rarely shifts his attention from what he is doing to look up when his mom calls his name. It seems as if he is more interested in objects than in people, and if he is looking at an interesting object, the social bid of a person doesn't capture his attention.

Attempting to Make Needs/Wants Known: Even before they develop words, young children have many different nonverbal strategies for getting their needs met. These include: directing their eye gaze to a caregiver and then to something they want, making sounds and looking at what they want, and reaching or using gestures to indicate they want something.

WHAT DOES WADE DO: Wade has an instinct for how to use his body, his face, and his voice to send messages to his caregiver. He may not integrate all these methods of communicating very well, due to his motor difficulties, but he clearly is attempting to communicate and will try a different strategy if the first one doesn't work.

WHAT DOES RYAN DO: Ryan seems not to understand what communication is and he rarely attempts to use his voice, eyes, face, or body to send clear messages to others. If he wants something, he usually tries to get it himself, or he may take another person's hand and use it like a tool to meet his needs—for example, by backing into his mom and wrapping her arms around him is a less-social way of requesting being held.

Attempting to Imitate: By around 12-14 months, most children will attempt to imitate simple motor movements and will play imitative games, such as pat-a-cake. They also imitate simple gestures, such as clapping and waving goodbye.

WHAT DOES WADE DO: Wade is socially tuned in and tries to match the behaviors of others. Even if his motor challenges compromise the precision of his hand movements, he tries to copy simple movements.

WHAT DOES RYAN DO: Ryan does not attempt to copy or match the behaviors of others. He resists attempts to participate in social games that involve simple imitative play.

Activities/Interests: One-year-olds play with cause-and-effect toys and enjoy sensory-motor play. They also play near other children and are usually receptive to the social approach of a familiar person, such as a brother or a sister.

WHAT DOES WADE DO: Wade is playing as one might expect in a one-year-old (simple cause-and-effect and other forms of sensory-motor play). He seems to be interested in and responsive to his sister.

WHAT DOES RYAN DO: Ryan is also playing in a sensory-motor way, but he may be less open to new activities than Wade. He tends to play on his own and is not very responsive to his sister when she tries to get him to play.

Preschool-Aged Children who Currently Function More Like 2½- to 3-year-olds

- Chronological Age: 4½ years
- Developmental Age: 32 – 36 months

Jacqueline: Child with Down syndrome without ASD. Jacqueline is an exuberant, delightful little girl who usually carries one of her dolls with her almost everywhere she goes. She speaks in 2- to 4-word phrases and sentences most of the time and consistently looks right at the person she is speaking to. It can be hard to understand her words, due to some articulation difficulties, but Jacqueline is quick to add gestures and miming motions to clarify her message. For example, she frequently uses a "come here" gesture of her right arm to recruit another child or adult to see her doll. She also shakes her finger at others, says "no, no, no," and frowns intently if she wants others to stop doing something. She loves books and story time and frequently stands up in circle time and directs a "shh" gesture to all of her children in the circle. She has an imaginary friend, who she talks to and directs others to greet.

Jacqueline tends to hug other children somewhat indiscriminately and can be unintentionally rough physically when intent on hugging a friend. If another child is sad or hurt, Jacqueline tries to comfort her by patting her back and saying "There . . . there . . . there. You sad." Jacqueline likes to play in the kitchen area during free play best of all, but she will also follow a friend to another play center. She seems to enjoy new experiences and expresses her enthusiasm by smiling and saying "cool" with an excited lilt to her voice.

Nora: Child with Down Syndrome and ASD. Nora is an independent, curious little girl who loves Buzz Lightyear and frequently says "tofinobeyo!" (which means "to infinity and beyond," a line from the *Toy Story* movies). Her words are directed to no one in particular as she runs and jumps and sometimes throws a toy. She doesn't seem to be aware that she could bump into someone else or accidentally hit them with her toy. Nora can talk in 3- to 4-word sentences, but most of her sentences were learned in chunks and come from scripts of her favorite movies or cartoons. She refers to herself as "Nora" and doesn't use pronouns such as "I" and "you" correctly. When she wants something, she says "Nora's turn."

It is often difficult to understand what Nora is saying and it is not always clear to whom she is speaking. When someone tries to understand and asks her to clarify, she usually walks away and doesn't add gestures or show others what she is talking about. She rarely tries to get another child to play with her and she rarely responds to another child's invitation to play, unless the game is tag, which she usually plays through one turn before wandering away from the game. She does not greet others. Nora loves to swing and will try to physically move other children from the swings to get a turn. Circle time seems to be her least favorite part of the preschool day and she frequently leaves the area or pushes other children who get too close.

WHAT TO NOTICE

In these two examples, we have a 4½-year-old child who is functioning more like a 3-year-old, so we want to think about the social and communication skills we would hope to see in a 3-year-old. In the example above, Jacqueline has many of the social-communication skills we would expect in a 32-to-36-month-old. These are described below.

Coordinating Eye Contact with Her Words: As spoken language develops, young children coordinate their eye gaze with increasing effectiveness and can use nonverbal cues to clarify their messages.

WHAT DOES JACQUELINE DO: Jacqueline consistently initiates and sustains a coordinated eye gaze with her listener when she is talking. Because she has difficulty with articulation, her listener may need additional nonverbal cues to understand her message and Jacqueline uses her eyes in a communicative way.

WHAT DOES NORA DO: Nora rarely looks directly toward the person to whom she is speaking. If her listener doesn't seem to understand the message, Nora doesn't use her eyes in a communicative way (such as looking at the person, looking at a desired toy, then looking at the person again).

Using Gestures, Voice Quality, and Facial Expressions to Support Verbal Communications: Children who are emerging talkers (i.e., using phrases and some full sentences comprised primarily of verbs and nouns, such as "I go swing"; "You eat pizza. Good?") frequently add gestures, alter their intonation patterns, and/or change their facial expression in order to punctuate their message, clarify their intention, and/or add emphasis or emotion.

WHAT DOES JACQUELINE DO: Jacqueline frequently adds descriptive or instructive hand movements to her words. Her gestures, though imprecise, carry emotion and she can convey the strength of her feeling by altering the speed or forcefulness of the movements. She changes the rate and rhythm of her speech, as well as her intonation patterns, when she is communicating for different reasons. For example, she raises her intonation and tips her head when asking if the food is good to the adult, indicating she is asking a question with clear, culturally learned gestures, vocal quality, and postures. She uses a clearly differentiated directive tone when insisting that her peers be quiet.

WHAT DOES NORA DO: Nora does not gesture spontaneously very often, either to clarify a message or to add emotion to it. Her voice tone doesn't vary, and she doesn't provide additional information in her facial expressions or changes in posture.

Showing Empathy for Others: Preschool-aged children begin to understand that other people have feelings and sometimes need help to feel better. Typically developing 3-year-olds usually notice when another child is sad or hurt and often make some attempt to comfort the person, particularly if he or she is a familiar person.

WHAT DOES JACQUELINE DO: Jacqueline appears to be very aware of other people's emotions, even labeling them spontaneously and trying to offer comfort when another child is hurt.

WHAT DOES NORA DO: Nora does not show awareness of other people's feelings. This lack of regard for others can look intentional, but usually reflects a basic lack of understanding that other people experience the world differently than you.

Spontaneity and Flexibility of Spoken Language: Preschool-aged children learn to use their words for a variety of purposes—to request something, to comment on it, to ask questions, to share information, to demand something, etc. They also generate new combinations of words, make predictable errors in grammar and syntax, and improve the complexity of their speech as they practice.

WHAT DOES JACQUELINE DO: Jacqueline communicates for lots of different reasons and puts together original phrases and verbal combinations.

WHAT DOES NORA DO: Nora tends to communicate for fewer reasons (usually to get a need met). She also seems to use phrases in chunks and many of her verbalizations are not spontaneous constructions she has created, but rather come from scripts in familiar books or movies. Nora also demonstrates some of the unusual language features that are associated with ASD, including: reversing the pronouns "I" and "you," calling herself by her own name, and reusing the same phrases over and over without clear regard for the context.

Social Quality of Initiations and Responses to Other Children: Children in the preschool years are developing appropriate social behaviors and learning how to behave in a variety of play scenarios. Children of this age learn to join others in play and invite others to play with them. They also begin to understand that sometimes you play a game longer than you might want to, and then you can switch the game to what you like best.

WHAT DOES JACQUELINE DO: Jacqueline frequently initiates towards other children and tries to recruit them to join her in her play interests. She also tries to participate in group games and responds to the social bids of her peers. She is an active participant in group instruction (circle time).

WHAT DOES NORA DO: Nora rarely initiates interactions with her peers and may respond to a play invitation, but only in a limited way (such as in certain games or only for a turn or two). She doesn't tend to persist in a game for the pure social enjoyment of playing, but abandons activities without communicating with her friends. Group instruction (circle time) is not an enjoyable learning venue for her and she does not seem comfortable when in close proximity to other children.

Elementary-Aged Children (Kindergarten – 5th grade)
Elementary School-aged Child Who Currently Functions Like a 2-year-old

- Chronological Age: 10 years
- Developmental Age: 18-30 months

Alicia: Child with Down Syndrome without ASD. Alicia is a fourth-grade student who spends most of her school day in a special education classroom with seven other children. She is accompanied by a teaching assistant to music, gym, recess, and lunch so that she can be with other fourth graders on a daily basis. Alicia is a quiet, shy, sweet-tempered child who is now in remission after treatment for leukemia. She has bravely endured a lot of medical procedures in her young life, and her health is improving. Alicia learned to walk when she was 4½ and continues to develop slowly, particularly in motor skills. She has low muscle tone and it takes her a little while to organize and initiate movement.

Alicia seems happiest when she is listening to music, sitting in the sun at the park, and being near animals. She has a therapy dog (Rocco) that comes with her to school, which has seemed to help her to adjust to being back at school after being in the hospital. The other children are interested in her dog and frequently approach Alicia to ask if they can pet him. Alicia smiles broadly when her peers approach her and she nods her head vigorously at their request. She communicates primarily through simple gestures and signs and can request food, Rocco, music, hugs, and outside. She is very affectionate, particularly with adults, and seeks being near an adult in most situations. She watches other children play, but rarely joins them on her own initiative. If an adult or another child who is familiar to her actively recruits her to join a game, she usually does so timidly, often showing more and more pleasure in the activity as it continues. When she listens to music, Alicia often rocks back and forth and smiles to those around her, giggling when her favorite parts are played. She is not interested in television, movies, or the computer, but can be very content sitting with a familiar adult and looking at picture books, particularly of animals.

Rose: Child with Down Syndrome with ASD. Rose is a fourth-grade student who also spends most of her time in the special education classroom. Attempts to include her with peers in activities such as music and gym have not been very successful, and Rose seems agitated when escorted to these classrooms. When her peers try to approach her or give her something (like a tambourine in music class), she turns away or walks away without really regarding them. Rose rarely smiles and often looks serious. Sometimes she laughs at unusual times, such as when someone is crying or gets hurt. She is very quiet and rarely vocalizes, unless she is very happy or very upset. Rose is physically very active and is rarely ill. She loves swinging, spinning in circles, and jumping.

Rose's educational team has been working hard to help her learn how to communicate basic requests, but Rose's responses are inconsistent. Sometimes she uses a sign to indicate "more"; however, the majority of the time she does not try to communicate. Rose likes to carry an object in each hand at all times and becomes distressed when her teachers try to get her to put the objects down to do an activity. Transitions between activities can be very challenging. During free play, Rose sits on the floor with her legs outstretched, rocks back and forth vigorously, while moving her hands rapidly in front of her face. Sometimes a teacher can get her interested in a three-piece puzzle or a cause-effect music toy, but usually Rose has difficulty initiating play with toys on her own.

WHAT TO NOTICE

Importance of Medical History: Some children with Down syndrome have a complicated medical history and have received extensive medical interventions. Sometimes, development is slower in children with health problems, either because of the illness itself or because of the learning opportunities the children miss during medical treatment. It is very important to consider a child's medical history when considering an additional diagnosis of ASD, as part of the criteria for autism involves ruling out any other possible explanations for the child's social, communication, and play behaviors.

WHAT DOES ALICIA DO? Alicia presents as a shy child with significant developmental delays, and her longstanding experience with medical treatment for leukemia poses challenges to her overall development. The chemotherapy she received has been associated with memory problems and she is often fatigued and not able to attend school. Understanding her history helps to clarify that there could be another explanation for her slow developmental progress.

WHAT DOES ROSE DO? Conversely, Rose is physically robust and healthy and her slow developmental progress cannot be attributed to illness.

Social Orientation. At a developmental age of two years, toddlers show awareness of others by watching them, smiling upon their approach, and seeking to be near them. These behaviors demonstrate that the child is engaged socially and is participating with others in a manner that is appropriate for his or her developmental level.

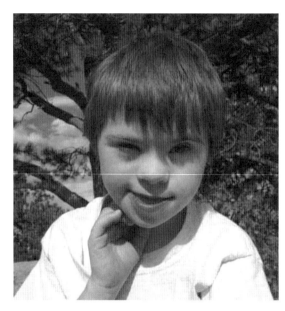

WHAT DOES ALICIA DO? Alicia shows interest in other children and responds positively when they come to her to ask about her dog. She seeks out being close to familiar people. Subjectively, she feels "connected" to adults and other children, even when she is not at the same skill level as the peers around her.

WHAT DOES ROSE DO? Rose does not appear to be interested in other children and tends to wander away when they try to interact with her. Being with her peers in a large group seems more distressing than pleasurable to her. She seems to act as if no one else is around and her attention is focused inwardly, as opposed to outwardly.

Attempts to Communicate. Developmentally, toddlers (one- to two-year-olds) are developing ways to communicate what they want, either through words, gestures, making sounds, or using their eyes. Even if their communicative efforts are hard to understand, young children who try to send messages to others understand the basics of social communication.

WHAT DOES ALICIA DO? Like other children of a similar developmental age (i.e., about 2 years), Alicia has learned how to indicate basic requests using nonverbal means (e.g., gestures or signs). Her vocabulary is small, but very useful to her and she sends simple messages to others frequently throughout the day.

WHAT DOES ROSE DO? Like other young children with ASD, Rose does not seem to understand the process of communication, and she rarely tries to send messages to others, either through verbal or nonverbal means.

Play Behaviors. Developmentally young children usually have relatively limited play skills and tend to seek out sensorimotor play (exploring the sensory features of objects and not yet developing play schemes). In fact, the sophistication of a child's play is thought to reflect his or her language ability.

WHAT DOES ALICIA DO? Alicia's interests are consistent with sensorimotor play; she tends to enjoy passive listening or sensory exploration and is not yet engaging in multistep play schemes. Her play skills reflect her overall receptive language ability.

WHAT DOES ROSE DO? Rose also tends to engage in sensorimotor play, although her preference is for high-intensity motor activities, such as swinging, spinning, and jumping. During toy time, she rarely shows interest in playing with objects, but rather engages in repetitive body movements.

Self-Soothing Strategies. One of the developmental tasks of early childhood is to develop strategies for coping with distress. Most young children seek comfort from others and find it calming to be near familiar people.

WHAT DOES ALICIA DO? Alicia seeks being close to familiar people, particularly when she is feeling shy or if she is in a new situation. She has the social instinct to trust others to care for her.

WHAT DOES ROSE DO? Rose does not rely on others for comfort; rather, she seems calmed by carrying objects or getting a lot of movement and stimulation. She does not seem to have the same sort of social affiliation or sense of trust and connectedness that Alicia demonstrates.

Elementary School-aged Child Who Currently Functions Like a 5- to 7-year-old

- Chronological Age: 10 years
- Developmental Age: 5 to 7 years

Porter: Child with Down Syndrome without ASD. Porter is a fourth-grade student who participates in general education classes and also spends time with a special education teacher throughout his school day. He likes being in his homeroom and always checks the job chart with enthusiasm each morning. He particularly likes the job of feeding the classroom's fish and sometimes he will feed them, even if it isn't his job. When Porter has decided he is going to add an extra feeding (which he knows is against the rules), he first looks around to see where his teachers are and tries to lift the top of the tank quietly. If he is caught and sent to the time-out chair, Porter cries and covers his face with his arm. When his time-out period is over, he often approaches the teacher, pats her back, and says "I sorry" several times and tries to hug her.

Porter likes the classroom routine, but can also be fairly flexible when changes in his schedule occur. He tends to "go with the flow." Porter's expressive and receptive language skills are lower than his classmates', and this sometimes frustrates him. However, he has learned that if he does not understand an adult's direction, he can watch what other kids do and follow their lead.

Porter plays a variety of games with other children during recess and play time. He likes to serve snacks to stuffed animals and will try to get others to join him in this game. Whenever he gives a stuffed animal a snack, he asks if it's good by looking right at the animal's face, holding both palms open in front of him in a questioning gesture, tilting his head, and raising his tone of voice at the end of the word in an inquiring manner. Then he appears to wait for a response from the stuffed animal, says "Yeah, yeah, yeah," and nods his head vigorously, sometimes rubbing his belly. Porter plays this way frequently and may repeat the same play scheme over and over and over, enjoying it each time.

Nathan: Child with Down Syndrome and ASD. Nathan is also a fourth grader. He learns best when there are fewer people around and he appears to be "in his own world" when in the general education classes with his peers. He is learning to greet people and responds to a visual reminder from his teacher to say "hi." He understands many of the classroom rules and likes predictable routines. He gets upset if he is not the Line Leader and will not readily participate in any other classroom job. When another child is Line Leader, he will physically put himself in that position and it can be difficult to redirect him to another place in line. Teachers have tried to prompt him to apologize after hitting another child, but he doesn't seem to understand what they want him to do, which confuses and upsets him.

Nathan's favorite activity is working on the computer and he has figured out how to get online and search the internet for his favorite websites. He also operates the DVD player and effortlessly finds his favorite section of a movie and replays it over and over. He likes to watch the credits of movies several times and becomes very distressed if interrupted before they are finished. Nathan is already showing some good reading skills and seems to have improved his talking as he became a better and better reader. Even though he has some very nice problem-solving and academic skills, he is not yet toilet trained during the day. He prefers the color yellow and gets upset if someone else gets an item of this color instead of him. When distressed, he is very difficult to console. Nathan doesn't sleep well and he only eats a few foods, including macaroni and cheese, chicken nuggets, and pizza crust.

WHAT TO NOTICE
Social Orientation: Thinking about Other People: During the middle childhood years, children become increasingly aware of other people's thoughts, feelings, and intentions. Children five years and older become more likely to change their behavior, based on what they think other people will think about it.

WHAT DOES PORTER DO? Porter is aware that his additional fish-feedings are against classroom rules and he has the social understanding to look around and make sure his teacher isn't watching when he tries to sneak the fish a snack.

WHAT DOES NATHAN DO? Nathan seems unaware of the thoughts and feelings of others in his classroom and doesn't often change his behavior spontaneously because of what others might be thinking. For example, his insistence on being Line Leader precludes him from considering how the "real Line Leader" might feel about his intrusion.

Social Conventions: Seeking reassurance and engaging in social conventions, such as greeting others and apologizing to someone you have annoyed, develops in early to middle childhood. Demonstrating knowledge of social conventions, and attempting to repair an interaction are developmentally appropriate social behaviors for elementary-aged kids.

WHAT DOES PORTER DO: Porter spontaneously greets others and initiates a routine for apologizing, which, although somewhat disingenuous (e.g., in the example above, we figure Porter will break this rule again and isn't truly sorry for feeding the fish), he does demonstrate knowledge of the social convention for apologizing and he attempts to repair the interaction. Even though feeding the fish is intensely fun, he also doesn't want his teacher to be mad at him.

WHAT DOES NATHAN DO: Nathan doesn't understand or enact basic social conventions, such as greeting others, saying "excuse me" when he bumps into someone, or apologizing if he hurts someone. This "unwritten" social code is not meaningful to him. His lack of social niceties is sometimes misunderstood by others as meanness, but he is actually completely unaware of many seemingly basic social conventions, such as greetings.

Developing Strategies to Help Cope with Language Problems: Children with communication difficulties, such as problems understanding complex language or challenges in pronouncing words clearly and consistently, often develop strategies to help them to function when their language challenges get in the way. If the child also has an ASD, the child is much less likely to develop and initiate some of the social learning strategies that can help—such as watching what other kids do and then doing what they are doing.

WHAT DOES PORTER DO? Porter has learned that when he doesn't understand what someone has said, he can look to see what other kids are doing and imitate their actions. This strategy has served him well in many new situations.

WHAT DOES NATHAN DO? Nathan does not seem to attend to the actions of other children and he is rarely seen spontaneously copying what they do—either in play or during school work. Instead of relying on imitation or looking to others to solve problems, Nathan usually tries to solve a problem by himself and either succeeds or abandons it.

Variety in Play: As children are learning a new skill, they will repeat it and repeat it until it is mastered. Some repetition, therefore, is adaptive and part of typical development. Children with a developmental delay of any kind are more repetitive in their play than children without a developmental disability. Therefore, some repetitive play is to be expected in children with Down syndrome, whether or not they also have an ASD.

WHAT DOES PORTER DO: Porter likes familiarity and routine and repeats the "feeding the animals" play scheme quite often. However, he is also open to participating in other activities and doesn't solely play in the same way each time.

WHAT DOES NATHAN DO: Nathan has limited play skills and also repeats the same activities on the computer over and over and watches the same sections of movies several times. It is difficult to interest him in novel activities.

Behavioral Flexibility: As children get older, they are challenged more and more to be flexible and to "go with the flow." Being adaptable to changes and managing transitions between activities becomes an age-appropriate skill that is necessary to accomplish before kindergarten.

WHAT DOES PORTER DO? Porter follows the classroom routine and moves between activities without additional interventions. He prefers certain toys but can usually accept a replacement. He may balk at some transitions, but overall is able to "go with the flow."

WHAT DOES NATHAN DO? Nathan becomes overly focused on certain events or activities (like being the Line Leader), has difficulty with transitions and unexpected events, and needs additional help leaving preferred activities, such as recess. He gets fixated on the color yellow and has a hard time being flexible and allowing another child to have something yellow.

Concluding Comments

Children with DS-ASD tend to have difficulties in core social relating and nonverbal communication that cannot be explained by their overall developmental level or past medical history. Specific behaviors tend to be associated with a co-occurring ASD, even though the exact form of these behaviors will differ, based on the child's developmental level. Please see Table 7-3 for a summary of behaviors that may be indicative of ASD in a child with Down syndrome. It is important to remember that a combination of several of these characteristics is necessary for diagnostic identification.

Implications for Intervention

One of the most important reasons for considering whether a child with Down syndrome is also presenting with an ASD is that often a qualitatively different approach to intervention is needed to promote development. Researchers continue to study the effectiveness of specific interventions for children with both Down syndrome and ASD. We offer some of our clinical impressions, based upon our clinical experience, in Table 7-4. It is our hope that future research will provide families and interventionists with an evidence base to draw from with regard to appropriate educational and therapeutic interventions for children with this complex combination of developmental disorders. In the meantime, a sys-

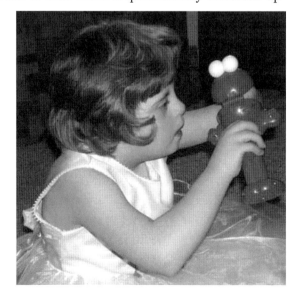

tematic approach to teaching, based upon developmentally appropriate targets and utilizing evidence-based practice in special education, is strongly recommended.

Table 7-3 Behavioral Tendencies Observed in Children with Down Syndrome and ASD

	Rarely	Occasionally	Frequently
Responds when his name is called	x		
Notices or regards others	x		
Greets others	x		
Tries to send basic communicative messages (verbally or nonverbally)	x		
Tries to imitate or copy the behaviors of others	x		
Shares emotions with others by directing facial expressions to other people in a moment of shared experience	x		
Responds to the approaches of another child	x		
Tries to continue a social interaction purely for the joy of being together	x		
Seeks comfort from others	x		
Shows a wide variety of subtle changes in emotions	x		
Expresses emotions that don't seem to match the situation		x	
Seems nonresponsive to pain		x	
Shows more interest in objects than people			x
Relies on his or her own exploration to solve a problem			x
Develops fixations on particular routines or rules and has difficulty being flexible with unexpected changes			x

Table 7-4 Suggestions for Intervention for Children with Both Down Syndrome and ASD

SOCIAL FUNCTIONING

- Directly teach pivotal social skills, such as sharing attention and emotion
- Facilitate social interactions with one peer at a time
- Focus on being socially responsive, following the child's lead and expanding the child's social interactions
- Find peer activities that minimize expressive language demands
- Educate peers about the child's strengths and challenges
- Provide opportunities to make choices

COMMUNICATION

- Implement a combination of parent training and direct child therapy
- Focus on developing nonverbal intentional communication skills
- Build in many opportunities to practice requesting—particularly in order to regulate another person's behavior (e.g., to get help, to get attention, to play)
- Use natural consequences to support requesting
- Teach different ways to request
- Teach waiting for request to be fulfilled
- Consider using basic sign language or other nonvocal forms of communication
- Assess receptive skills and teach to the receptive level of child
- Think about how communicative intervention can support positive behaviors

POSITIVE BEHAVIOR SUPPORTS

- Conduct functional behavior assessments and intervene in light of function
- Create a daily checklist in the child's home-school book to communicate about risk factors for problem behaviors (e.g., sleep, illness)
- Consider teaching communication skills as an adaptive alternative to problem behavior
- Create back-up plans for days where child's behavior is disregulated

LEARNING STYLE

- Minimize distractors when teaching a new skill
- Provide frequent practice performing a new skill correctly
- Use visual supports
- Establish predictable routines
- Consider computer-based instruction
- Reduce memory demands
- Embed teaching in natural situations to enhance generalization

Acknowledgments

Understanding Down syndrome and autism is a community effort. Many thanks to the families who participated in our studies and have been very generous with their time, effort, and wisdom.

With appreciation to our colleagues at JFK Partners, the University Center for Excellence in Developmental Disabilities at the University of Colorado Anschutz Medical Campus; specifically Cordelia Robinson, Ph.D., Carolyn DiGuiseppi, Ph.D., Nancy Lee, Ph.D., Amy Philofsky, Ph.D., and Audrey Blakeley-Smith, Ph.D. Our collaborations with Dr. Lisa Miller of the Colorado Department of Public Health and the Environment and Sarah Hartway have been instrumental in shaping our interest in this area.

The leaders of the Down Syndrome-Autism Connection (specifically Margaret Froehlke, Robin Sattel Zaborek, Lorri Park, and Sarah Hartway) have been instrumental in keeping the work going and helping us to find relevant ways to share it.

Recommended Resources

Websites

- Autism Society of America: www.asa.org
- American Academy of Pediatrics: www.aap.org/healthtopics/autism.cfm
- Centers for Disease Control: www.cdc.gov/ncbddd/autism
- National Down Syndrome Society: www.ndss.org
- National Down Syndrome Congress: www.ndsccenter.org

Books about Identifying Children with Autism

Chawarska, K., Klin, A., Volkmar, F.R., & Powers, M. (2010). *Autism Spectrum Disorders in Infants and Toddlers: Diagnosis, Assessment, and Treatment.* New York, NY: Guilford Press.

Stone, W.L. & DiGeronimo, T.F. (2006). *Does My Child Have Autism? A Parent's Guide to Early Detection and Intervention in Autism Spectrum Disorders.* San Francisco, CA: Jossey-Bass.

Books about Interventions for Children with ASD

Gray, C. (1993). *The Original Social Story Book.* Arlington, Texas: Future Horizons.

Harris, S.L. & Weiss, M.J. (2007). Right from the Start: Behavioral Interventions for Young Children with Autism. 2nd ed. Bethesda, MD: Woodbine House.

Koegel, R.L. & Koegel, L.K. (Eds.) (1996). *Teaching Children with Autism: Strategies for Initiating Positive Interactions and Improving Learning Opportunities.* Baltimore: Paul Brookes.

Prizant, B.M., Wetherby, A.M., Rubin, E., Laurent, A.C., & Rydell, P.J. (2006). *The SCERTS Model: A Comprehensive Educational Approach for Children with Autism Spectrum Disorders.* Baltimore: Paul Brookes.

Quill, K.A. (2000). *Teaching Children with Autism: Strategies to Enhance Communication and Socialization.* New York, NY: Delmar Publications.

Rogers, S.J. & Dawson, G. (2010). *Early Start Denver Model for Young Children with Autism: Promoting Language, Learning, and Engagement.* New York, NY: Guilford Publications.

Schopler, E., Mesibov, G.B., & Hearsey, K.A. (1995). Structured teaching in the TE-ACCH system. In E. Schopler & G.B. Mesibov (Eds.), *Learning and Cognition in Autism.* New York, NY: Plenum Press.

Simpson, R. (2005). *Autism Spectrum Disorders: Interventions and Treatments for Children and Youth.* Thousand Oaks, CA: Corwin Press.

Please address correspondence to: susan.hepburn@ucdenver.edu; or Susan Hepburn, Ph.D., JFK Partners, Dept. of Psychiatry and Pediatrics, University of Colorado Anschutz Medical Campus, 13121 E. 17th Ave., Box C234, Aurora, CO 80045.

References

American Psychiatric Association (2000). *Diagnostic and Statistical Manual of Mental Disorders – Fourth Edition, Treatment-Revised.* New York, NY: APA.

Autism and Developmental Disability Monitoring Network (2006). Prevalence of autism spectrum disorders – United States. *Morbidity and Mortality Weekly Report: Surveillance Summaries 58* (SS10): 1-20.

Berk, L.E. (2009). Infants, children, and adolescents. 3rd ed. Boston: Allyn & Bacon.

Fombonne, E. (2005). Epidemiology of autistic disorder and other pervasive developmental disorders. *Journal of Clinical Psychiatry 66 (SUPPL 10):* 3-8.

Sparrow, S.S., Cicchetti, D.V., & Balla, D.A. (2005). *Vineland Adaptive Behavior Scales.* 2nd ed. San Antonio, TX: Pearson Publishing.

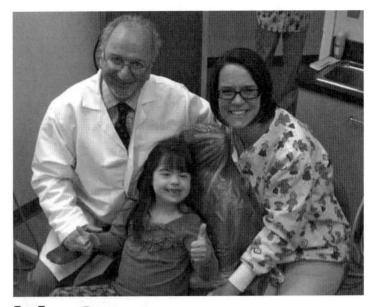

8

Oral Health Care
Finding the Way for a Child with Down Syndrome-Autism Spectrum Disorder

David A. Tesini, DMD, MS, FDS, RCSEd, and Kristi Seibel, DMD

Introduction

"I lost my Roadmap to good oral health care . . . is it time to get out my GPS?"

A vast amount of information is available and awaits us at every turn, in all media forms, and in every contact we have with our healthcare providers. Books, pamphlets, articles, booklets, the Internet, newsletters, blogs, tweets. . . . all provide access to oral health knowledge. We read about infant oral care, brushing and flossing, the importance of periodic dental visits, diet and nutrition, protection of teeth while playing sports, early orthodontic treatment of crooked teeth, the importance of fluoride—and the list goes on and on. We've seen pictures of severe gum (periodontal) disease, malocclusions, and broken teeth, websites direct us to dental offices that provide services to our children, articles tell stories of unmet dental needs in the special patient populations, and about how to deal with insurance companies and the financial restraints put on both the patients and providers. These anxieties often become the *real barriers* to dental care for Children with Special Health Care Needs (CSHCN).

Complicating these barriers is the parental anticipation of poor cooperation. Don't be nervous or afraid to bring your child to the dentist because you're thinking that your child will be hard to deal with and the "experience will be a disaster." Don't procrastinate! It will most likely be harder the longer you wait.

If only we could back the car out of the garage, get on the right road, pull into the parking lot of the dental office, get out of the car, head toward the neon sign that reads "get same-day dental care here," stroll back to the car, and exit the parking lot with perfect "pearly whites." The typical dental journey for CSHCN, however, sends you in so many directions that when you come out of the house, you can't even find the *road* to the dental office parking lot, much less get the care that your child needs. What can you do?

This chapter will give you a plain and simple understanding of the *GPS (Great Parenting Skills)* you will need to advocate, navigate, and access the dental care needed for your child with a Down Syndrome-ASD diagnosis. Good oral health requires discipline, and parents and caregivers alike need only to understand five simple areas:

1. Understanding the Oral and Dental Findings in DS-ASD
2. Developing Your Philosophy: Start Looking for a Dentist Now
3. Early Infant Oral Care: Understanding the Importance of Daily Oral Hygiene
4. Overcoming the Behavior Barrier: The D-Termined™ Program of Repetitive Tasking
5. Advocating as Part of the Team

Understanding the Oral and Dental Findings

Both children with Down syndrome (DS) and autism spectrum disorder (ASD) have some specific dental and oro-facial findings. These two diagnoses may coexist but they need not be compounding. That is, there need not be extra complications just because your child has both conditions.

Dental Characteristics Associated with Down Syndrome

The dental oro-facial characteristics of individuals with Down syndrome have perhaps been studied more than those of any other syndrome group. Facial characteristics of individuals with DS are usually definable and predictable for the dentist. We know that the maxillary (upper jaw) is small in relationship to the mandible (lower jaw) and is often described as an "incomplete development of the midface complex." The tongue is often protruding due to hypotonia (low muscle tone) and has been described as being "relatively large" in comparison to the small maxillary arch (palate). Often the airway is compromised by related medical conditions such as dry and thickened mucous membranes or anatomic blockage of the airway by large tonsils and/or adenoids, which can result in mouth breathing. Orthodontic characteristics include anterior open bites and posterior and anterior crossbites consistent with a small upper jaw and a protruding lower jaw.

Primary teeth are often retained for years longer than is typical, and often permanent teeth (the upper permanent lateral incisors) are missing. Researchers have found a high prevalence of periodontal and gingival (gum) disease and low prevalence of dental caries (cavities) in children and adults with Down syndrome. Causes include impaired cell mediated immunity to infections, altered salivary chemistry, specificity of bacteria colonization (the actual bacteria in the mouth can be different), abnormal and delayed eruption of both the primary and permanent teeth, malocclusion and abnormalities of dental alignment (crooked teeth), poor oro-myofunction, inadequate oral hygiene, bruxism (grinding), mouth breathing, and even vascular capillary arthrosclerosis.

Other systemic factors such as immune-competency, poor circulation, and general physical deterioration combine with environmental factors to influence oral and dental disease susceptibility. These same factors can influence the way the jaws grow and the teeth come in.

Behaviorally, many children and adults with Down syndrome are genuinely warm and honest, but they often become stubborn and resistant, which can complicate dental treatment.

Dental Characteristics Associated with Autism

Although dental conditions in children with ASD are less remarkable (and certainly less defined), there are some generalizations that can be made. Food consistency, texture, taste, and temperature have effects on the diet of children with ASD. Sweets, sometimes used in conjunction with behavior modification programs, may contribute to caries (cavity) development. In most studies, however, children with autism have been reported to have a comparable (cavity) index and cavity level as children without autism. Tongue coordination difficulties, oral tactile sensitivities, side effects of medications they may be taking, bruxism, and food pouching may lead to additional dental problems.

In the past, some reports had pointed to a concern that an increased prevalence of esophageal reflex in children with ASD might cause dental erosion (wearing and loss of enamel) in both the primary and permanent teeth. Recent research (Mourisden et al., 2010) found no evidence for increased GI diseases, but toothwear may still exist. Increases in dental trauma have also been reported due to "accident proneness" and self-inflicted behaviors, but these findings have not been substantiated.

Children with ASD frequently have difficulties cooperating with dental procedures in the office, as well as dental care at home due to impairments in social interaction and communication skills, sensory and tactile responses, and repetitive patterns of behaviors.

Dental Characteristics of Individuals with DS-ASD

So, with the understanding of some of the dental findings in Down syndrome and autism, is it just a matter of combining both to arrive at a characteristic dental picture of children with DS-ASD? Well, most likely no! The reason for this hesitancy is that, to date, there has been no dental research on the dental conditions of patients with DS-ASD. We do know, however, that *for all children* behavior and lifestyle variables affect dental conditions. The behavior characteristics of the DS-ASD group may be specific enough to provide environmental differences that are not seen in children with Down syndrome or autism spectrum disorder alone.

Developing a Philosophy: Start Looking for a Dentist Now!

To start: you should find a dentist who is familiar with treatment of CSHCN. Although availability is limited in some areas, a pediatric dental office is a good place to start. Ask your neighbors and friends, your pediatrician, relatives, and school contacts

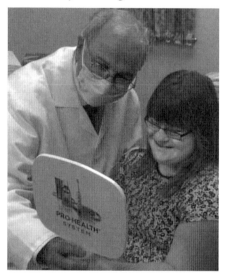

to recommend a dentist who might best be able to treat your child with special needs. Remember, the capabilities of the ancillary staff (the dental assistants and dental hygienists at the dental office) are just as important as the training and experience of the dentist.

Open a dialogue with the dentist and staff. Ask the dentist about his recommendations and experience in treating individuals with disabilities and how you as the parent/caregiver can aid in the process. Encourage dentists not to look at autism or Down syndrome as a "disorder," but instead to understand that the challenges and different behaviors lie in the "perspective" in which these children view their world. Perhaps it would be better to change the name from autism spectrum disorder to autism spectrum perspective (ASP). For us as pediatric dentists, it becomes less about *managing* the behavior and more about *understanding* it.

Many children with Down syndrome characteristics will develop jaw growth and tooth alignment problems early in life. Although recognized by dentists and parents, these malocclusions are often left untreated simply because the child is "handicapped." Lack of orthodontic treatment often magnifies the underlying disability. Remember, the only reasons for not recommending orthodontic treatment for a child with DS-ASD is poor oral hygiene and/or unmanageable behavior. **Having a developmental disability is not a contraindication to receiving orthodontic treatment.**

Once you find a dental office and prior to your child's first visit, you should ask your child's doctor(s) if there is any important medical history to tell the dentist or if your child needs antibiotic premedication. Some dentists find it helpful to have a medical history to review prior to the first visit. If any questions arise, the dentist may even consult with the physician ahead of time, so that there is no delay on the day of the appointment. Additionally, on that first contact with the dentist's staff, let them know about your child's behavioral, social, and educational characteristics. Details, which only you as a parent can provide, can help the dental staff understand your child. No one else knows your child like you do!

Early Infant Oral Care and the Importance of Daily Oral Hygiene

Here is a very good way to understand caring for your child's teeth, especially one with a diagnosis of DS-ASD:

> *Think of a single tooth. When it first peeks through the gum, it doesn't know whose mouth it is coming in to …"Will I be kept clean?" it may ask… "will I be crowded?… or what kind of food will I eat?" It doesn't know that it has now made a permanent home in the mouth of your special needs child.*

Early infant oral care is important for all children, and especially so for children with SHCN. The Surgeon General's Report of 2000 identified that CSHCN are at increased risk for oral diseases. (U.S. Dept. of Health and Human Services, Oral Health in America). The first dental visit in infancy, the *"age one dental visit"* (American Academy of Pediatric Dentistry), is simply the first step on the Roadmap to Good Oral Health Care.

Before going any further, we must understand how dental decay (cavities) form in the first place. In an effort to simplify a truly complex process we will use the following formula:

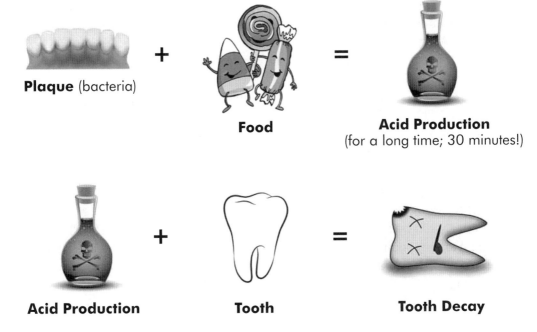

Plaque (bacteria) + **Food** = **Acid Production** (for a long time; 30 minutes!)

Acid Production + **Tooth** = **Tooth Decay**

The same formula applies for gum disease (gingivitis and periodontitis). At the most basic level, it can be thought of as a bacterial disease that occurs slowly over a long period of time.

Your child's dentist will of course explain much more, and can evaluate your child's cavity risk with a tool called CAMBRA (Caries Management by Risk Assessment). They can test the acidity (pH) of the saliva, review daily snacks, the family history of dental problems, and even the role that "crooked" teeth might play in causing dental disease. Additionally, they will be able to identify any risk factors for gum disease.

Prior to that first visit, there are some steps you can take to get on the road to good oral health care that are applicable to *everyone*. Let's call it:

Basic "Dentistry for All"

We all know sugar is bad for your teeth, but that is only part of the story. Remember the other factor in the cavity equation—*time;* specifically how often and how long food particles stay in the mouth. This is why sticky foods such as fruit leathers or dried fruit can be a big problem (they take a long time to "melt away.") Starchy foods can also form a sort of gluey mass that sticks to teeth—remember making paper mâché? It was flour and water. Fresh fruits and vegetables or hard cheeses are a better alternative for snacks. Additionally, frequent snacking provides a near constant source of debris in the mouth that can lead to decay. Whenever possible, it is best to try to limit between-meal snacks. Likewise, nighttime bottles and sippy cups allow milk, formula, or juice to be present for many hours, often causing cavities even before all the baby teeth erupt!

Cleaning the mouth should start even before the first tooth erupts (around six months). A washcloth or burp cloth can be used to wipe out your child's mouth and remove debris. When the first tooth erupts, a soft bristled toothbrush can be introduced. The bristle should be placed on the tooth, angled down towards the gumline, using a small circular scrubbing motion to clean.

As your child grows, she may be able to take over the brushing, first with "hand over hand" brushing with a toothbrush and then with only parental observation and guidance. A manual toothbrush is fine, but if there is any concern regarding fine motor skills, a motorized brush (when properly used) can be helpful.

Toothpaste comes in a variety of flavors and textures; some experimentation may be needed to find one that is acceptable for your child. Use only a smear of toothpaste on the brush if your child cannot yet spit well. Young children should have a pea-sized amount of toothpaste. Flossing is recommended for areas where the teeth are touching. Floss holders can aid in the task.

Teeth should be brushed twice a day, because bacterial plaque forms every 8 to 12 hours. Flossing should ideally be done once daily, particularly if there is any contact between the teeth. The earlier the routine is established, the greater chance of success.

Your child's dentist can help. If it is too overwhelming for you to introduce the brush and floss, perhaps a prescription mouth rinse or a different process could be recommended that would help while your child is learning the other hygiene skills. Don't lose heart before the trip even starts.

Remember that good oral health care is a journey. Some of you reading this chapter may look at those last paragraphs and think, "Well, we're heading in the right direction" and that is great! But for those who are thinking "Nice idea, but we'll never get there!" please know that slow, small steps can still get you there—it just might take a while. Find one thing that seems like it might work for you and try it. *Be determined to succeed!*

Overcoming the Behavior Barrier . . . The D-Termined™ Program

In a word, *behavior* is often the greatest barrier to receiving quality comprehensive dental care for children with DS-ASD. Impaired receptive and expressive language skills, impairment in social interaction, dyspraxia, and stereotypic repetitive behavior patterns are not only distracters in the education and social environment, but also present problems in the dental office. Recognizing this problem, a group of researchers (Marshal, Sheller, et al.) looked at the predictors of patient cooperation for dental patients with autism. Of particular interest were the facts that:

- Children 6 years and older who could not read were more uncooperative for their dental appointments.
- Children who were 4 years of age or older and who were not toilet trained were more likely to be uncooperative for the dentist.
- Having a concurrent diagnosis with autism was associated with uncooperative behavior, but taking medication was not associated with uncooperative behavior.
- Children who were unable to sit still for a haircut were also always uncooperative for the dentist.
- Only 40 percent of children who could brush their teeth at home were uncooperative, whereas those who needed to have a parent brush their teeth were almost always uncooperative for the dentist.

It is interesting to note that in this study repeated visits alone (without a road-map) would not necessarily improve patient cooperation. This is surely counterintuitive to what *we* would expect, right? We would suggest to you that a random, unstructured, problem-focused, interspersed dental visit cannot provide the structure necessary for familiarization to benefit in improving the behavior. Dental care should be provided through a structured and defined approach, such as in the *D-Termined™ Program of Familiarization and Repetitive Tasking.* This is a non-pharmacological technique of managing children's behavior at the dental office that may improve treatment success.

The D-Termined™ Program of Familiarization & Repetitive Tasking: For Parents and Dentists

The D-Termined™ Program is based in applied behavior analysis (ABA) theory and uses the "Familiarization through Repetitive Tasking" philosophy so often used

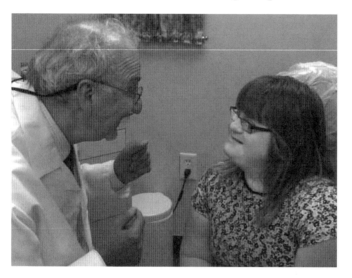

in education programs for children with ASD and Down syndrome. The D-Termined™ Program encourages us to understand that the most important factor in being successful is to "be determined." There are many cases where the severity of the DS-ASD diagnosis, combined with the scope of needed dental treatment, would require immobilization devices, sedation, or general anesthesia. Although several factors enter into the decision, no factor is as important to the success of the nonsedative behavior guidance approach as the willingness of the dentist and the parent to "try, try, and try again."

If you watch the D-Termined™ program DVD (see Suggested Resources), you will learn that there are three repetition factors that are the keys to success.

1. *Eye Contact ("look at me")*

    This must be mastered by the patient and practiced by the parents at home between visits.

    Difficulties with eye contact are a characteristic feature of the autistic behavior pattern. It is almost like the children want to look at you but can't. They want to look at you but they need to be reminded…. They want to look at you but they need to be directed. One way you can initiate eye contact is by a visual cue. Hold your fingers in the "victory sign"—point to the child's eyes and then pull your hand and fingers toward your eyes.

2. *Positional Modeling ("put your feet out straight and hands on your tummy")*

    "Feet out straight"—Whenever the knees are up and feet are flat footed on the seat of the chair, the kids tend to want to "push off," which results in uncontrollable and unmanageable movements. Position their feet out straight, and, if necessary, stabilized by holding above the knee for a ten-second count. (Stabilizing a patient to support him or her in position for ten seconds or less is not considered restraint.)

"Hands on your tummy"—This serves two purposes:
1. it provides sensory input that the hands are in contact with something (in this case, the stomach), and
2. with the hands down low, the dentist will have a longer reaction time to compensate for "hand grabbing" or hand/arm resistance.

3. *Counting Framework ("1, 2, 3, 4, 5, 6...")*

You can make it verbal and visual by using picture stories or counting charts in conjunction with counting.

Once mastered, these repetitions can be used in the five major components of the D-Termined™ Program. Notice that *all* components begin with the letter "D."

- 1ˢᵗ: Divide the skill into small components.

    Coming into the operatory, sitting in the chair, putting chair back, sitting in the chair with feet out straight and hands on tummy. Count finger, count fingers, count tooth, count four upper front teeth, count teeth, etc. A total of 20 steps are identified in dividing the tasks needed for a classic "first" visit. (See the Behavior Management Report at the end of the chapter.)

    Each step becomes a separate objective instead of a means to an end. Some parents create a customized visual aid to mark the completion of each "step" of the visit for their son or daughter.

- 2ⁿᵈ: Demonstrate the skill.

    Positional modeling means that you take a skill, such as "legs out straight" and you actually put the legs out straight and then support that position for a 10-second count. Follow immediately after every 10 count with praise. Continue with "hands on your tummy," meaning position the hands on the tummy and support that position with a 10-second count, followed immediately with praise...and so on for all the 20 steps

- 3ʳᵈ: Drill the skill

    Schedule a series of 5-6 repetitive visits one week apart. Use the task list to divide up the tasks and skills to be mastered and customize to each patient.

- 4ᵗʰ: Delight the repetition

    Everyone in the operatory remains happy, upbeat, and determined to keep trying.

- 5ᵗʰ: Delegate the patient to your trained auxiliary

    Each weekly visit is scheduled for 30 minutes (may take more, may take less). THIS MUST NOT BE DENTIST TIME INTENSIVE. A trained dental auxiliary (assistant or hygienist) will start each visit and move the procedure along the step progression. The dentist will then come in at the end and start the last "rerun"—from putting the chair down to the point on the task list that is the objective for the day. The bulk of the Repetitive Tasking must be done by the auxiliary or it will become either too expensive for the parents or a financial burden on the dental office. Behavior guidance techniques MUST NOT BE DENTIST TIME INTENSIVE.

Practice with the parents or the teacher between visits is very helpful. Send them home with a disposable mirror, saliva ejector, and fluoride trays. Do not revert to the varnish. The purpose of using the trays is to help the child acquire the skill to have tastes, impression trays, and various other materials in the mouth. It is for desensitization in preparation for impressions, mouthguards, radiographs, orthodontic retainers, and appliances.

And one last word for the dentist . . .

This technique should not be time intensive for the dentist, but it *is* time intensive for the staff. All staff should be trained in the D-Termined™ Program but only some of your staff will actually "get it." That is, only some staff will have the proper voice tone and rhythm and the proper timing to be directive to both the patient and parent at the same time, and inherently know the right holding and touching pressure. This can't be taught, and somehow comes from within. Some of your staff will "get it" and can get into their DS-ASD patient's world, whereas other staff members will have a harder time trying to get the technique to work for them.

The D-Termined™ Program of Familiarization and Repetitive Tasking will be a welcomed addition in your Behavior Guidance Armamentarium. Watch the DVD with your staff at lunch some day. Keep in mind four words that will help ensure your office's success with the D-Termined™ Program: *"Get into their world."*

Advocate as Part of the Team

"Yes! The dentist needs your help."

Parents need to do their part. First, keep your appointments. So many times breakdown in the patient/doctor relationship occurs because patients (parents) do not take seriously keeping appointments and being timely. The dentist has organized his daily schedule to accommodate all his patients. You may even want to call first thing in the morning and offer to come in a little earlier or later if the doctor would like. If not, "we'll see Jimmy at 11:00 as planned."

Remember, the dentist and his staff are part of your service and support team. Bear in mind that your own past experiences may have created some negative attitudes that will only hamper the dentist's efforts at treating your child. Be open to suggestions and opinions that may vary a bit from your own. Can you imagine a child with a cavity whose parent says, "I don't want the fillings done because it will be too traumatic" versus a parent who says, "how can we work together to successfully get the fillings done"? Which scenario do you think is most likely to achieve a lifetime of good dental health?

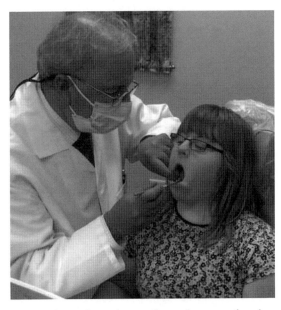

Providing the dentist with pre–appointment information about your child is critical, because as we said before, it is less about *managing* the behavior and more about *understanding* it. Let the dental staff know: What is your child doing at school? How is that going? Is she using picture boards, story books, or sign language? What is it like when she has a meltdown? What sensory issues does your child have, especially around the face and mouth?

Start early…be disciplined…and be part of the dental team. The reward will be in your child's smile for a lifetime. And you will always be able to find your way—even without the GPS.

Suggested Resources

- *D-Termined™ Video* available on YouTube at: www.youtube.com/watch?v=artQFqd6osQ
- American Dental Association website, "Public Resources" section: www.ada.org
- American Academy of Pediatric Dentistry website, "Parent Resource Section": www.aapd.org
- National Institute of Dental and Craniofacial Research, information specific to individuals with special needs: www.nidcr.nih.gov/OralHealth/Topics/DevelopmentalDisabilities/PracticalOralCareOverview.htm

Behavior Management Report

Patient: _____ Age: _____

Diagnosis: _____

Parent: _____

School Contact/Support: _____

Repetitive Tasking for D-Termined™ Visits

Date: _____

	1	2	3	4	5	6

Into Operatory
Onto Chair
Sitting in Chair
Legs Out Straight
Hands on Tummy
Chair Back Down
Chair Back Up
Raise Hand to Stop
Mirror Exam

Mirror & Explorer Exam
"Mr. Thirsty / Ms. Issippi"
Prophy Cup (plain)
Prophy Anterior Teeth w/Paste

Prophy Posterior Teeth w/Paste
Floss

Toothbrush F (taste)
Empty Fluoride Trays
Brush On Flouride Anterior Teeth

Maxillary Flouride Tx w/Tray
Mand Flouride Tx w/Tray
Other (specify)

Time Units (15 minutes increments)

Tesini Pediatric Dentistry & Orthodontics, 410 Boston Post Road, Sudbury, MA 01776

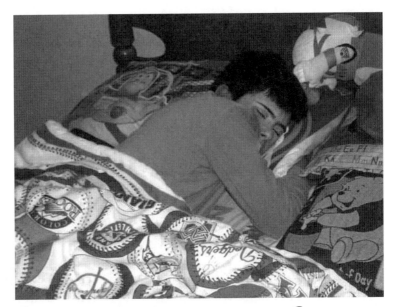

9

Behavioral Treatments for Sleep Problems in Individuals with DS-ASD

Terry Katz, PhD, and Ann Reynolds, MD

Parents often assume that sleep difficulties are "part of life," especially if they have a child with co-occurring diagnoses of Down syndrome and autism spectrum disorder (DS-ASD). In some respects, this is correct. Many families of children diagnosed with ASD do experience difficulties with sleep, and some evidence suggests that children with DS-ASD have an even greater incidence of sleep difficulties than do children with Down syndrome alone. However, while it is common for children with DS-ASD to have a sleep disturbance, this does not mean that sleep problems are insurmountable. On the contrary, there are a number of strategies that may improve a child's sleep.

It is hard to overestimate the importance of good sleep; improvements in sleep often lead to improvements in physical and emotional health as well as potential improvements in attention and learning. We are continually learning more about the consequences of poor sleep. Difficulties with sleep have been linked to poor physical health, including the risk of obesity, diabetes, and heart disease. Children with DS-ASD may be particularly at risk for health difficulties that are tied to poor sleep. A lack of sleep affects our ability to remember information, concentrate, make good decisions, and process information.

The impact of poor sleep persists over time. A lack of adequate sleep is called a "sleep debt," and studies show that we do not get used to or adapt to insufficient sleep. The longer we go without adequate sleep, the worse we perform on tests of cognitive functioning. Sleep also affects our emotional state. Research indicates that poor sleep is related to depression, anxiety, and hyperactive behavior. Further, there is evidence to suggest that better sleep may result in positive behavioral changes during the day such as improvements in activity level and attention. Some research even suggests that sleep promotes the processing of negative experiences in a helpful way.

Sleep Basics

Knowledge of the mechanics of sleep will help you understand the basis for effective strategies that improve sleep. While our understanding of sleep is not complete, researchers have learned a great deal about how we fall asleep, what happens while we are sleeping, and what to expect as we grow and develop. Scientists have used this information to identify problems in sleep and ways to promote healthy sleep.

While researchers have learned a great deal about sleep, there is still much to learn. We have some knowledge about what happens when we don't get enough sleep, yet we lack a complete understanding of why we actually sleep. Until scientists were able to measure electrical current in the brain (in the 1930s), it seemed impossible to study what happens when we sleep. Studies using electroencephalograms (EEGs) have shown that sleep is divided into two major states: Non-REM and REM sleep. REM stands for rapid-eye movement sleep. Non-REM sleep is also called "quiet sleep" or "slow-wave sleep."

What Happens during Sleep

When we first start to fall asleep, we experience a stage called "alpha sleep." During this stage we are still awake, but relaxed and calm. This relaxed wakefulness sets the stage for non-REM sleep, which consists of four stages that involve deeper and deeper sleep:

- *Stage 1* of non-REM sleep typically lasts only a few minutes and is a light sleep. Our body temperature drops, we become more relaxed, and we are easily roused.
- We then move to *Stage 2.* During this stage we are firmly asleep, but we are also easily awakened. Approximately half the night is spent in Stage 2 sleep, and this phase usually occurs during transitions to other sleep stages.
- *Stages 3 and 4* are referred to as deep sleep or slow-wave sleep. During deep sleep, our breathing slows, our temperature drops even more, and it is much more difficult to wake up. Researchers have determined that deep sleep is a time for body renewal and repair. When

we are sleep deprived, we typically move into the deeper stages of sleep quickly and spend more time in these stages. Researchers have interpreted this to mean that deep, slow-wave sleep helps us feel restored and refreshed.

We typically move through one or two cycles of non-REM sleep before moving into REM sleep. While non-REM sleep is described as "quiet" and includes a slowing of bodily functions, REM sleep is "active." Rapid eye movement is characteristic of REM sleep, and this is the time when we dream. Our breathing and heart rate increase and are similar to the rates we experience when we are awake. Surprisingly, the part of our body responsible for the "flight or fight" response is twice as active during REM sleep as it is when we are awake. While our mind is quite active, our body is hardly moving; in fact, muscles that are not needed for breathing, eye movements, or hearing are basically paralyzed during this stage of sleep. There is some indication that REM sleep may enhance learning and memory. We enter REM sleep about three to five times a night or approximately every ninety minutes. People who have repeatedly been awakened from REM sleep do not do as well at learning a new task as those who are repeatedly awakened from non-REM sleep. There is thus some evidence to suggest that REM sleep promotes our cognitive and emotional well-being, while non-REM sleep promotes our physical well-being.

Throughout the night we move through the different stages of sleep. Some changes occur in the length of a full sleep cycle and in the amount of time we spend in each stage as we grow and develop. Most of our deep sleep occurs in the first half of the night, with longer periods of REM sleep occurring during the latter part of the night. As we move from one stage to another, we experience changes in our brainwave patterns. It is not unusual to move about and shift in our bed during these transitions; we may also briefly awaken and make sure that "all is well." Such arousals occur most frequently when we are moving in and out of REM sleep. These changes in arousal and brief awakenings occur in all children and adults, and they are not considered interruptions in sleep unless we cannot return to sleep afterwards. For many individuals, this is a time when some sleep disturbance may occur, and an awareness of this process may point to effective ways to improve the quality of one's sleep.

The Typical Sleep/Wake Cycle

In addition to understanding what happens while we sleep, it is useful to look at what helps us actually fall asleep at night and be awake and alert during the day. There are two physiological or biological mechanisms that control our sleep/wake cycle: circadian rhythms and homeostasis.

Circadian Cycles: Circadian comes from the Latin phrase "about a day." We all have biological cycles that occur approximately every twenty-four hours. In addition to our sleep/wake cycle, a wide number of other biological functions have a daily rhythm; some of these physiological processes involve body temperature, the release of hormones, digestion, and elimination. These processes work in concert to move us through the sleep and wake cycle. For example, we typically fall asleep when our body temperature drops, and we wake up as it starts to increase. The production of various hormones, such as melatonin and cortisol, has also been linked to our sleep/wake cycle.

Our circadian cycles are all somewhat longer than twenty-four hours, lasting closer to twenty-five hours in length. This tendency toward a twenty-five hour cycle is one reason why it is easier to stay up later than it is to fall asleep earlier than our natural sleep time. There are a number of cues, however, that promote a twenty-four hour cycle. Sleep researchers call these cues zeitgebers, which means "time givers" in German. Some zeitgebers include light, social demands, and ambient temperature. Exposure to light in the morning and darkness in the evening helps us maintain a twenty-four hour cycle. For this reason, individuals who are blind have circadian rhythm disturbances and sleep problems. A decrease in temperature is another signal that it is time to go to sleep. Social cues also keep us on a twenty-four hour schedule. We respond to cues from others about our sleep/wake cycle. When we are with people who are sleeping or getting ready for bed, we sense a need to do the same.

Homeostasis: In addition to circadian rhythms, we also have homeostatic drives. These drives help us maintain a physiological equilibrium and explain why we typically eat when we are hungry or drink when we are thirsty. We all have a homeostatic drive to sleep, and we become sleepier after an extended period of wakefulness. The longer we are awake, the stronger our drive to sleep becomes. We also experience a drive to sleep when we have accumulated a sleep debt.

Ideally, our homeostatic drive and circadian rhythms work in concert to keep us awake and alert during the day and asleep at night. Knowledge of our homeostatic drive for sleep and circadian rhythms provides a basis for understanding why we might have trouble falling asleep at certain times. For example, the hour before our regular bedtime is often called the "forbidden zone" because it is extremely difficult to fall asleep during this time. Even though our sleep drive is strong, our circadian rhythms make it difficult to fall asleep. For the same reason, it is hard to fall asleep in the morning following a night of little or no sleep.

How Do I Know Whether My Child Has a Sleep Problem?

Determining whether your child has a sleep problem is not always as clear-cut as it may seem. Different people need different amounts of sleep. Some of us are truly "short sleepers" who need less sleep than the amount typically recommended and others are "long sleepers" who need more. Furthermore, our sleep needs change as we grow and develop. A young child, for example, needs more sleep than an adolescent. One way to determine if someone is getting enough sleep is to examine their behavior during the day. Are they sleepy or tired during the day? Do they fall asleep at unusual or inconvenient times? Is it hard for them to awaken in the morning? Do they have behavioral difficulties (such as hyperactivity or irritability) that might be explained by a lack of sleep? Answering these questions helps us determine whether or not a child has a sleep problem.

We also need to consider an individual's preferences for bedtime and wake time. Some people naturally tend to be early risers (larks) while others naturally become energized late in the evening (owls). There are also developmental differences; for example, adolescents tend to prefer later bedtimes. It also appears that children with autism spectrum disorders may need less sleep than same-age children with typical development.

Some sleep habits may pose more difficulties for parents than for children. A young child might not be at all upset about needing to fall asleep with a parent by his or her side, but this may cause difficulties for his or her parents. The same may be true for the length of time it takes a child to fall asleep and the time at which he or she wakes up in the morning.

Some of the first questions that parents and professionals should ask when assessing a child's sleep include the following:

- Does your child maintain a regular sleep schedule (school and nonschool days)?
- How long does your child sleep each night on average?
- Does your child have any problems at bedtime?
- Does your child have any problems falling asleep?
- Does it take your child more than 20 to 30 minutes to fall asleep at night?
- Does your child snore or have any problems breathing during the night?
- Does your child have seizures that are not well controlled?
- Does your child have any unusual/repetitive behaviors during the night?
- Does your child need assistance to wake up in the morning?
- Does your child seem sleepy or overtired during the day?
- Does your family have a history of sleep problems?

If the answers to these questions lead to any cause for concern, see the next section on assessing a child's sleep difficulties.

How Are Sleep Problems Formally Evaluated?

There are a number of ways that sleep problems are evaluated. The first step should always be to obtain a thorough medical history and physical exam from your child's physician or primary care provider in order to determine whether there may be a medical cause for any sleep difficulties.

Medical Evaluation: There are many medical problems that may affect sleep, including issues that cause pain or discomfort. These include gastroesophageal reflux, constipation, abdominal pain and other gastrointestinal concerns, hunger, wheezing/coughing, seizures, eczema/itchy skin, headaches, dental pain, and joint pain. Medications that the child is taking need to be considered, as some medications make it more difficult for a child to fall asleep at night. It is necessary to determine whether asthma, sinusitis, allergies, or nasal congestion are affecting sleep and whether a child is snoring or gasping for breath at night. This may indicate that a child is experiencing poor air movement/oxygenation while sleeping. This may cause fragmented sleep, which has physical and behavioral implications.

Snoring and breathing issues are especially important to assess when evaluating children with DS-ASD because of the prevalence of disordered breathing while sleeping in children with Down syndrome. There is mounting evidence that disordered breathing while sleeping has a negative impact on daytime behavior and attention. (Please see the section on Sleep-related Breathing Disorders below.) A thorough medical history will also include questions about nutrition; there is some evidence to suggest that low iron stores may be related to restless leg syndrome or periodic limb movement disorder. Finally, psychiatric conditions including anxiety and depression should be ruled out, as they can contribute to difficulty sleeping. Please see Chapter 4 for more details about medical conditions that might affect sleep in individuals with Down syndrome and ASD.

Sleep History: After a comprehensive medical evaluation has been completed, the next step is to obtain a good understanding of a child's sleep history. This includes learning about the development of the child's sleep habits. Has he always had difficulty sleeping or is this a new problem? When did the difficulties begin? Did they coincide with changes in the child's environment, family situation, schooling, daily routines, or with age? Learning about the child's daily routines, amount of exercise, exposure to outdoor light, dietary habits, dinner routine, and evening schedule is helpful. Noting if, when, and for how long he naps should also be considered, as well as whether he ever falls asleep while riding in the car, at school, or during other activities. Specific information about bedtime routines, aspects of the bedroom environment, and what happens after parents say "goodnight" is essential and thus needs to be reviewed. Parents are often asked to complete sleep diaries that document when a child is put to bed, when he falls asleep, how often and how long he is awake during the night, and when he wakes up in the morning. Information about daytime activities, naps, and use of medications are also frequently noted in a sleep diary.

Sleep Study: For many children, this is all the information that is needed to assess their sleep difficulties and develop an effective treatment plan. For other children, further assessment is needed. If there are concerns that medical conditions may be affecting sleep, children may need to complete an evaluation in a sleep laboratory. Ideally, this will occur in a medical facility that has experience evaluating children. A sleep study or polysomnogram (PSG) provides information about how long a child takes to fall asleep, how much sleep he or she gets during the night, progression through the sleep stages, whether sleep apnea is present (and if so the severity), whether periodic limb movements occur while the child is sleeping, and whether there are any EEG abnormalities that might suggest the presence of seizures.

Preparation for a sleep study involves placement of electrodes and sensors on an individual's head, face, and body that allow monitoring of movement and physiological functions. Many children with DS-ASD are able to successfully complete a sleep study with little difficulty; other children need time and careful preparation before entering a sleep laboratory. For those children, the use of Social Stories, desensitization to specific aspects of the sleep study (such as wearing electrodes), and creative use of distracters and tangible rewards may help children successfully complete these studies.

Try to become familiar with what will occur during your child's study prior to arriving for the appointment. If possible, visit the sleep lab and learn about each step. You may want to develop a picture schedule to prepare your child for what will occur. You can then anticipate any potential difficulties and work with the sleep study team to develop a successful plan to help your child. For example, you can determine where you can be while your child falls asleep and what bedtime activities might be acceptable. While we would not recommend strategies such as co-sleeping to help a child fall asleep at home, we want to do whatever we can to make the sleep study a success. Some children will need extra time to practice (and become desensitized to) specific aspects of the sleep study.

Be patient and know that with time your child should be able to tolerate this procedure. During desensitization or an actual sleep study, some children respond well if they can see their parents undergoing some of the same procedures. Other children like to practice by putting electrodes on their dolls or stuffed animals. Maintain a calm and positive attitude while practicing the steps of a sleep study as well as during the procedure itself. Make sure your child has had plenty of exercise or activity during the day of the scheduled sleep study; having less sleep and being more tired may make it easier for your child to fall asleep and stay asleep throughout the night.

Sleep Problems and Intervention Strategies

Parents of children with autism spectrum disorders and Down syndrome report that their children demonstrate a range of sleep-related problems, including difficulty falling asleep, going to bed at a late time, sleeping for only a short amount of time, frequent night waking, and early morning rising. Other difficulties commonly noted include sleep-disordered breathing, teeth grinding, parasomnias, restless sleep, and daytime sleepiness. While these concerns cover a wide range of sleep difficulties, they do not include all sleep problems that may be encountered. The International Classification of Sleep Disorders is used for diagnosis and coding of sleep problems, and includes over 80 different sleep disorders. We will limit the discussion in this chapter to sleep difficulties that are commonly reported by parents of children with autism spectrum disorders and Down syndrome.

Difficulty Falling Asleep at Bedtime

Difficulty falling asleep at bedtime is a common problem experienced by many children, especially those with autism spectrum disorders. For these children, it often takes 30 minutes or more to fall asleep. Bedtime is often characterized by resistance or refusal, frequent curtain calls ("can I have one more drink of water . . . pleeease!), and a long time settling. For many families, these difficulties are frustrating and chronic.

Going to Bed Late

Going to bed at a late time often occurs when a child has difficulty falling asleep. Parents report that their children do not seem sleepy and often fall asleep much later than they, the parents, would like. A variety of techniques may be effective in helping children fall asleep with less difficulty. A number of these techniques also address other sleep problems that we will discuss subsequently. These strategies are often referred to as "sleep hygiene" because they promote healthy sleep. Many of the strategies that we discuss in this chapter were developed by Beth Ann Malow, MD, MS, Neurologist and Director of the Sleep Disorders Program and Burry Chair in Cognitive Childhood Development of Vanderbilt University, Nashville, Tennessee, and her colleagues as a product of the Autism Treatment Network (ATN), a program of Autism Speaks and the Autism Intervention Research Network on Physical Health (AIR-P).

Daytime Activities

The first step toward improving sleep is examining daytime habits and making changes that may promote sleep at the end of the day. The main areas we examine include exercise, light, food, daytime sleep, and bedroom use.

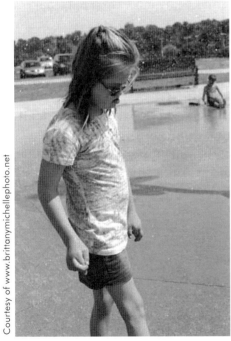

Courtesy of www.brittanymichellephoto.net

Exercise: Parents should encourage their children to get plenty of exercise early in the day. Among its many benefits, exercise promotes healthy sleep. Exercise should not, however, occur too close to bedtime, as physical activity is often stimulating and actually makes it more difficult to fall asleep. It is best to move toward calming and relaxing activities at least an hour before bedtime.

Light: Children should be exposed to as much light as possible during the day. Exposure to daytime light (especially natural light) suppresses our melatonin levels and primes us to respond well to a decrease in light as evening falls.

Food: Caffeine acts as a stimulant that promotes alertness and interferes with sleep. Take time to look at the foods that your children are eating to make sure that they are not getting caffeine late in the day. While most of us realize that coffee and dark sodas contain caffeine, others may not realize that it is also present in chocolate and some clear drinks. A careful inventory of foods that may contain caffeine may therefore be informative.

Caffeine remains active in our bodies for long periods of time. The half-life for caffeine in adults is approximately six hours. This means that if someone drinks a beverage that contains 100 milligrams of caffeine, they will still have 50 milligrams in their body six hours later. The exact half-life of caffeine in children is not known, but some researchers hypothesize that it may be longer for children. Overall, it is best to avoid caffeine altogether in children, but it should definitely be avoided after noon if at all possible. If it is hard to cut caffeine out of your child's diet, consider diluting caffeinated beverages with water or a noncaffeinated drink.

Daytime Sleep: when thinking about daytime habits, consider the timing of naps for children who still take them. Generally, naps should be completed by 4:00 in the afternoon in order to avoid a later bedtime.

Bedroom Use: Take a look at how your child's bedroom is being used during the day. In order to promote strong sleep associations, we recommend that a child's bedroom only be used for sleep. The use of a child's bedroom for time-out may result in negative and anxious associations, while the use of a child's bedroom for play may result in excited and playful associations. When a bedroom is only associated with sleep, it is easier to fall asleep. If it is not possible to keep a bedroom only for sleep, try to make sure that the bed itself is reserved for sleep and physically mark an area of the bedroom that is reserved for play.

Evening Activities

Evening activities also play a role in regulating a child's sleep. Moving toward calming, relaxing, and relatively easy activities in the hour before bed is advisable. Try to avoid roughhousing and intense physical play before bedtime. In fact, avoid any activities that are stimulating and exciting. For instance, a favorite behavior such as watching a portion of a movie repetitively can also be over stimulating and interfere with going to sleep. It may be necessary to rearrange schedules so that these fun activities occur at other times during the day.

Routines: Developing set routines in the evening also promotes successful sleep. Try to keep the lights down low and avoid exposure to light, as this might decrease melatonin levels. Melatonin is a sleep-promoting substance that is released by the brain. Its release is inhibited by light. When thinking about light at bedtime, remember that television, video games, and computer monitors all emit bright light that may interfere with sleep.

Sleep Environment: The child's sleep environment should also be considered. Is his bed and bedroom comfortable? The following factors should be considered when evaluating whether your child's bedroom is helping or hindering sleep.

Lights should be off if possible, but some children do need a night light. Some children have developed routines in which they have become used to having an overhead light or desk light on while they try to fall asleep. Families may find that using light bulbs with progressively lower wattage may decrease their children's dependence on light at night. Also consider the output from hall lights and digital clocks.

Sounds should be kept to a minimum. Think about where your child's room is placed relative to the rest of the household. Is your child able to hear distracting or potentially stimulating noises? If so, it may be beneficial to move his bedroom to a quieter, less central location. Some children respond well to the use of a "noise machine," which produces calming white noise or nature sounds that mask distracting household noises. If a noise machine is used, take care that it stays on so that there is no change in the child's sleeping environment throughout the night.

Tactile sensations should also be considered. Try to attend to your child's preference for certain textures in bedding and pajamas. Children also respond to different amounts of pressure on their body. While some children might prefer little input, others are comforted by deep pressure. Many children respond well to the use of a weighted blanket or a sleeping bag. When using weighted blankets, take care to ensure that the material in the blankets cannot be removed by a restless child.

Consistency: Consistency is the basis for good sleep. Try to keep daytime, evening, and bedtime routines the same whenever possible. While today's busy families cannot always maintain a consistent schedule, it helps, for example, to have dinner at the same time every evening. If possible maintain the same bedtime and wake times every day of the week, including weekends. Avoid varying bedtime and wake times by more than one hour. The more consistent our daily schedule, the more our bodies and minds become conditioned to expect sleep to begin at a certain time and respond accordingly.

Families should carefully consider when to put their children to bed. If possible, keep track of when your child tends to actually fall asleep (versus when the child is put to bed) and how much sleep he or she gets each night. Some children with autism spectrum disorders may not need as much sleep as other children their age, and going to bed too early may be counterproductive. They may also have biological clocks that tend toward a late bedtime. Finally, avoid putting a child to bed during a time that has often been referred to as the "forbidden zone." This is the time during which we are all more alert and have great difficulty falling asleep. A child who has been struggling to fall asleep may fall asleep more readily when bedtime is moved to a later hour by avoiding this period of alertness. Once good bedtime routines and sleep behaviors have been established, it is often possible to gradually move the bedtime to an earlier time.

Once children are in bed, they need to fall asleep independently. Make sure that anything your child uses to fall asleep at the beginning of the night will be available throughout the night. You may recall that earlier in this chapter we discussed the fact that we all go through brief periods of arousal throughout the night. If nothing changes after falling asleep at the beginning of the night, we should have no difficulty remaining asleep throughout the night. If, however, changes do occur, it is much more likely that we will become alert during these brief periods of arousal. Thus, in addition to falling asleep on their own, children should fall asleep in the same place that they will sleep throughout the night. Children who are allowed to fall asleep in one place (such as the couch or a parent's bed) and are then moved to their own bed later in the evening often wake up during the night.

Calming Activities: Consistent bedtime routines are a cornerstone of good sleep. An effective bedtime routine lets children know that it is, in fact, time for sleep. A bedtime routine should consist of a small number of calming and easy activities that prepare a child for sleep. Look carefully at the activities that typically occur before bed and determine whether these activities should be part of an actual bedtime routine. For example, bath time is often calming for children, but some children react negatively to this. Think about ways to make bath time less aversive or move bath time to an earlier time in the day. There are a number of sensory strategies that may make some bedtime tasks (such as teeth brushing and bathing) less stressful.

Visual Schedules: Many children with autism spectrum disorders respond positively to the use of visual schedules at bedtime. A visual schedule depicts the activities involved in a bedtime routine. If, for example, a child's bedtime routine includes brushing teeth, bath time, putting on pajamas, and singing songs, a visual schedule would include a picture for each of these activities. Parents may use photographs, picture icons, or written lists to represent each activity. Some children also respond well to the use of objects rather than pictures. We recommend teaching children to learn to move through their schedule on their own with support from their parents. Try to keep the visual schedule in a central location.

Bedtime routines should take approximately thirty minutes or less and involve only a few activities. The idea is to gradually move closer and closer to the bedroom and to engage in progressively relaxing and sleep-promoting activities. A visual schedule increases the consistency and predictability of bedtime routines and may thus reduce a child's anxiety. Use of visual schedules also promotes independence and mastery. There are a number of resources that teach parents about using visual schedules. An excellent resource for this is the Autism Speaks website (www.autismspeaks.org).

Relaxation Techniques: Many children resist falling asleep on their own. They may be anxious, afraid of the dark, or have significant separation anxiety. In addition to the sleep hygiene suggestions that we have already outlined, an anxious child may benefit from bedtime relaxation techniques. These simple techniques include taking deep breaths or alternately squeezing and relaxing one's muscles. Some children may learn to do this by practicing being a "toy soldier" versus a "rag doll." You might think of other ways to convey the idea of tightening and then relaxing one's muscles. Other children may benefit from a massage or sensory techniques such as joint compression. As is true for many of the techniques that we describe, some trial and error may be necessary to come up with a calming routine for your child.

Helping Your Child Fall Asleep Alone

Children who have become dependent on sleeping with another person may be particularly resistant to learning to sleep alone. A variety of strategies may be effective. Some parents will try the "cold turkey" or "crying it out" approach. Parents who use this method decide that they will say good night to their children and then leave the room with the expectation that their children will fall asleep on their own. Parents

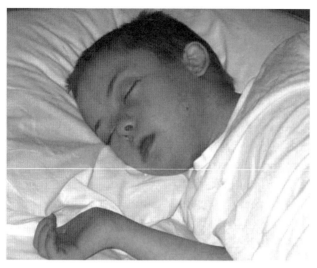

who use this method resolve not to return to their children's bedroom "no matter what." While this approach is often effective and efficient, it is emotionally difficult for many parents and children. Fortunately, it is not the only way to teach children to sleep independently. A number of more gradual approaches work well for many families.

Basically, these approaches involve saying goodnight and leaving the room, but allow parents to periodically check in with their children if they are distressed. The goal is to gradually increase the length of time between visits and to keep all interactions "brief and boring." Children may also learn to fall asleep independently without their parents leaving the room. Parents may stay near their children's bed (without any physical touching) while their children fall asleep. The plan is for parents to gradually move farther and farther away from their children's bed until they are out of the room. All of these methods will work, and it is often beneficial to pair progress in learning to sleep alone with rewards in the morning. These may include engaging in a special activity, or earning stickers or a small present.

Co-sleeping (when parents and children sleep together) is a family decision, and we respect parents who have made this choice. Many families, however, have resorted to co-sleeping as a way of helping their children get some sleep and would actually prefer to have their children sleep in their own beds. Teaching children to sleep alone in their own beds in a separate bedroom from their parents involves the same gradual approach discussed above. Parents may gradually move their children farther and farther away from them in the family bed and then have their children sleep in a bed near them. The child's bed may then be gradually moved to another bedroom.

It is often easier for parents and children to start this process by moving together to the child's bedroom and for parents to then move farther and farther away from their child. Few children object to this initial change (as long as they are still sleeping with their parents). Following this plan requires more transitions for parents but fewer transitions for children. For those families who are not sure whether they want to continue co-sleeping, it may be helpful to remember that all of us tend to sleep better, and with fewer interruptions, if we sleep alone rather than with another person.

Responding to Night Wakings

Teaching children to fall asleep on their own and in a consistent location also minimizes night wakings. This is a common problem for children with autism spectrum diagnoses. In addition to helping your child learn to fall asleep independently, you should develop a plan so that you have a consistent way of responding if your child wakes up during the night. If feasible, talk with your child about your expectations for sleeping through the night. Visual aids (such as a stop sign on the door) may be useful, and Social Stories are another effective technique.

You should respond to your child's distress (especially if he is anxious), and doing so before he becomes more upset is advisable. You should also, however, take care to ignore the inconsequential shifting and stirring that takes place during the night. It is fine to comfort a child who needs reassurance, but as with all interactions that occur after you say "goodnight," they should be kept to a minimum.

The **bedtime pass** is another technique that helps with night waking and difficulties falling asleep independently. This is a technique that was developed by Patrick Friman, Ph.D., and his colleagues. The bedtime pass is a small card that has an attractive picture on one side and the words "bedtime pass" on the other. When children are given this card at bedtime, they are told that they will receive a reward if they still have the pass in the morning. Children who do need to talk with or see their parents during the night will need to forfeit their pass (and a reward) for that night. Using a meaningful picture (including a picture that represents a child's special interest) on the pass may be quite effective; some children become attached to the pass itself because of the strong positive value attached to the picture. Some children benefit from using more than one pass when they first start this program.

Changes in your response to your child's night waking or sleep resistance may result in your child actually getting worse before he gets better. This is also true if you make changes to how your child falls asleep (especially if you stop sleeping with your child). Know also that after your child spends some time testing to make sure that there isn't anything he or she may do to change the situation ("maybe if I just keep crying . . ."), the situation will improve. If your child is getting up at night, be sure to consider safety issues. All doors and cabinets should be locked, and any dangerous materials should be kept well out of reach. It may also be necessary to put a bell on your child's door so that you will be alerted if he leaves the bedroom.

Early Morning Awakening

Early morning awakening is different from waking in the middle of the night and then returning to sleep at some point. Some children wake up earlier than their parents would like because of their need for less sleep. If that is the case, letting children stay up later at night may result in a later wake time. Eliminating naps for children who still take them may also delay the start of the day for some children.

Some children simply need less sleep and are ready to go much earlier than their parents. These children need to learn how to entertain themselves safely and quietly. Parents and children can work together to develop a morning schedule and a basket of toys and activities for morning time. Some children also respond well to visual cues about when they are allowed to go to their parents or other family members. A

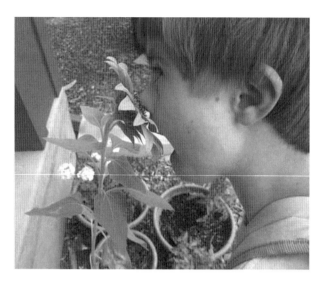

light with a timer may be used to cue children that it is permissible to leave the room only when the light is on. Parents may be able to gradually set the timer to go off at later times in the morning. Rewards for playing quietly and staying in one's room are often effective as well. As always, safety issues should be considered. As early morning awakening may be a sign of depression, a child's mood should be assessed if this represents a change in behavior.

Nightmares

Nightmares are common and typically occur during REM sleep and in the later part of the night. When children wake up from nightmares, they will typically remember at least part of what they have dreamt. Stress and anxiety have been linked to an increase in nightmares, so helping children learn to relax and be less anxious through simple relaxation techniques often results in fewer nightmares. It is advisable to provide some comfort to children who awaken from bad dreams, while helping them return to sleep in their own bed. Try not to spend too much time talking about your child's nightmare during the night and maintain a calm and matter-of-fact attitude.

Parents should try to maintain the sleep routines that have been established. Try to stay calm and do not provide too much reinforcement for having woken up in the middle of the night. It is not always necessary to talk about the nightmare the next day, and it is often best to avoid putting too much emphasis on a child's nightmare. If you do need to talk with your child about the nightmare, try to keep the conversation short and to the point. For children who have difficulty expressing themselves verbally, drawing pictures may be a valuable technique. If a child's nightmares persist, think about what might be upsetting for your child and try to address these issues well before bedtime.

Parasomnias

Parasomnias are common in childhood and tend to run in families. Some children cry out during the night but are not actually awake. These children may be experiencing night terrors, which are also called non-REM parasomnias. Other types of parasomnias include sleepwalking, sleep talking, and confusional arousals. Night terrors and nightmares are often confused with one another, but are actually quite different and respond best to different strategies.

Night Terrors: Night terrors are characterized by loud, piercing screams. Children experiencing night terrors are not actually awake. Night terrors typically occur during the first third of the night and are more common during the deep sleep phases of non-REM sleep. Children do not respond to attempts to provide comfort during these times. In fact, children may appear more agitated if others try to interact with them during a night terror. Remember that children are actually asleep during these episodes even if they seem awake and they usually do not recall much, if anything about the incident. If they remember anything, it is typically a single image but not a dream sequence. Some of these images may be quite frightening to a child and may include monsters or dangerous people. The fact that children are usually moving during these episodes tells us that they are not in REM sleep (when almost all movement is suppressed) and are not, in fact, dreaming. There is some evidence to suggest that night terrors are more common in younger children; they frequently stop by the time a child enters adolescence.

Confusional Arousals: Confusional arousals are another type of parasomnia. Children frequently sit up during these episodes and appear to be in a confused state. At times, forcing a child from a confusional arousal may result in some aggressive behavior. These types of arousals usually occur in children under the age of five and are similar to night terrors in that the child typically does not remember the event. Sleep walking is fairly common in school-aged children and is more common in boys than in girls.

Reacting to Parasomnias: There is some evidence to suggest that sleep fragmentation and sleep deprivation may increase night terrors. Noises or movement nearby may also be triggers. Improving a child's sleep routines may thus decrease the frequency of night terrors. During the time a child is experiencing a parasomnia, ensure his safety, but do not awaken him or try to stop the event. Even if your child is sleepwalking, all you need do is help him or her get back to bed and provide comforting, soothing statements. Although parasomnias may improve with age and better sleep hygiene, be sure to let your physician know about these difficulties. In some instances, parasomnias are an indication of medical issues, including nighttime seizures, so it is important to discuss your child's night terrors with a physician.

Teeth Grinding: Some sleep researchers consider teeth grinding, or sleep-related bruxism, to be a type of parasomnia. It is not clear what causes teeth grinding. Stress and anxiety may contribute to teeth-grinding, so relaxation techniques may reduce this behavior. There is also some indication that dental problems and the shape of the jaw may contribute to this problem, so consultation with a dentist is often advised. Dental guards or splints (if tolerated) decrease teeth grinding and lessen the physical impact of this behavior.

Delayed Sleep Phase Disorder: As children transition to adolescence, they commonly begin to develop later bedtime schedules and consequently experience delays in their circadian rhythms. Good sleep hygiene practices help these adolescents maintain typical sleep schedules. In more extreme cases, an individual may develop a delayed sleep phase disorder (DSP). If allowed to follow their own preferences, children with DSP will fall asleep late at night and then sleep until late in the morning.

They do not experience any difficulties falling or staying asleep as long as they are able to follow their own schedule. Thus, if there are no pressing reasons to change the schedule of an individual with DSP, treatment is not necessary. Most children, however, do need to conform to a traditional school and work schedule.

Treatment for delayed sleep phase disorder involves gradually and systematically changing a child's bedtime. Light therapy and some medications may also shift a child's sleep schedule. If you are considering these strategies, it is essential to talk with a healthcare professional who is skilled in treating DSP. Incorrect timing of light therapy may, for example, lead to a worsening of a child's sleep schedule.

Narcolepsy

Narcolepsy is an uncommon sleep disorder that involves excessive daytime sleepiness. While many think of this disorder as occurring in adults, it has been diagnosed in children as young as five years of age. Individuals with a diagnosis of narcolepsy will have extreme and sudden urges to sleep. They may suddenly fall asleep at any time during the day, even while they are eating, talking, or engaging in positive interactions. A tell-tale sign of narcolepsy is *cataplexy.* This involves the loss of muscle control during the day and often occurs during times of intense emotions, including positive emotions. Children with narcolepsy may also evidence temporary paralysis as they fall asleep or when they are first awakening.

Diagnosis of narcolepsy involves a nighttime and daytime sleep study. Currently, there is no cure for narcolepsy; treatment involves medication and good sleep hygiene. At this time, we don't know whether narcolepsy is more common in children with DS-ASD than it is in other children.

Sleep-Related Breathing Disorders

Sleep-related breathing disorders are some of the most common difficulties for children with DS-ASD. The incidence of obstructive sleep apnea (OSA) in people with DS is significantly higher than in the general population. Obstructive sleep apnea (OSA) is a serious disorder that has important behavioral and medical implications.

In brief, individuals with OSA have a narrowing of the airways, which makes it difficult to breathe during sleep. This can cause levels of oxygen to drop while levels of carbon dioxide increase. These changes (difficulty breathing as well as changes in levels of oxygen and carbon dioxide) result in disrupted sleep as the individual awakens and gasps for air. Once the individual has obtained enough good breaths, he returns to sleep. This happens repeatedly throughout the night, resulting in poor sleep and sleepiness during the day. This in turn may lead to difficulties in activity level, attention, memory, processing speed, and learning as well as other behavioral problems. The changes in oxygen and carbon dioxide levels are also physically stressful and may lead to heart and lung issues.

Parents may first become concerned about their child's sleep because of behaviors they notice during the night. A child with OSA may snore, gasp for breath, or sleep with his head tilted up or in an odd position in an attempt to improve breathing. If parents notice these difficulties, they should consult with their child's physician to determine whether a sleep study is indicated. Diagnosis of OSA is confirmed with polysomnography.

For many individuals with OSA, treatment may involve medication, surgery (removal of the tonsils and/or adenoids), or use of a device that provides positive airway pressure. This device provides air pressure to keep the airway open. Individuals wear a mask that connects via a hose to the machine that provides the pressure. One of the most common devices used for people with OSA is continuous positive airway pressure (CPAP). Respiratory technicians teach individuals how to use the device.

Learning to wear a mask and use the machine may be initially challenging, but children with DS-ASD are able to learn to use these devices. Graduated exposure and desensitization techniques have been quite effective. It is often best to take a gradual approach in which children first learn to wear a mask without any airway pressure and then slowly learn to tolerate longer and increased amounts of pressure. Other strategies that have been effective include decorating masks or having other family members wear them as well. Children may be given masks before they have been evaluated for OSA so that they can begin the desensitization process. This is an effective strategy for children with DS-ASD since these children are particularly likely to require the use of a positive airway pressure device at some point in their lives. The use of continuous airway pressure has been linked to less fragmented sleep and improved learning, behavior, and physical health.

Rhythmic Movement Disorder

Rhythmic Movement Disorder is characterized by repetitive motion of the head, trunk, or limbs, including head banging and rocking. It usually occurs during the transition from wakefulness to sleep. Rhythmic Movement Disorder is most often seen transiently in infants and toddlers but may persist in children with autism and other developmental disabilities to older ages. No specific treatment is indicated, but padding your child's sleep environment may be helpful.

Restless Legs Syndrome/Periodic Limb Movements in Sleep

Restless Legs Syndrome (RLS) is a sensorimotor disorder that involves an urge to move the legs, typically occurs at bedtime, and is associated with an uncomfortable sensation. RLS can be associated with difficulty falling asleep. *Periodic Limb Movements in Sleep (PLMS)* are defined by repetitive stereotypic movements of the limbs during sleep. *Periodic Limb Movement Disorder* (PLMD) includes PLMS but is also associated with insomnia or daytime sleepiness.

RLS has been reported in about 2 percent of children and is challenging to diagnose in children with difficulty communicating symptoms. A polysomnogram is necessary for making a diagnosis of PLMS or PLMD. Iron deficiency has been associated with RLS and PLMD in adults and children. Identification and treatment of iron deficiency in children with sleep disorders may be considered, although more research is needed to determine the efficacy of this intervention.

Medical Treatment

Once underlying medical issues have been addressed and a good behavioral plan is in place, medications are sometimes prescribed if the child is still having difficulty falling asleep and remaining asleep.

Treatment with melatonin has been found to be helpful in treating insomnia in children with ASD. Melatonin is a hormone that is produced in the brain. Melatonin production is suppressed by light, but as light is dimmed, melatonin levels increase. Increased doses of melatonin have been linked to drowsiness, and melatonin has been used to reset people's biological clocks.

While studies have not supported the use of melatonin to treat sleep disorders in children with typical development, melatonin appears to be safe and effective (at least in the short term) in individuals with an intellectual disability. (Some studies included children with ASD. Melatonin secretion has been noted to be low in small studies of children with ASD.) However, there are no studies in children with Down syndrome.

Synthetic melatonin is available as a dietary supplement and should always be used along with good sleep routines. It is important to discuss the use of melatonin or any other supplement with your physician before use. Other medications such as clonidine are often used to treat insomnia but no appropriate studies have been completed.

Conclusion

We would like to conclude this chapter by emphasizing the importance of good sleep. In our research and clinical work, we have seen the ways in which poor sleep affects mood, behavior, and the ability to learn. We have learned a great deal from the families with whom we have worked and we have been encouraged by the changes that we have been able to accomplish by working with them as a team. We have seen how addressing children's sleep difficulties can significantly improve their lives and the lives of their families. Parents of children with DS-ASD should remain optimistic that with proper intervention their children's sleep will likely improve.

Reading List

- Autism Speaks. (2012). AIR-P/ATN Tool Kit. Strategies to improve sleep in children with autism spectrum disorders: A family and clinician tool kit. www.autismspeaks.org/family-services/tool-kits.
- The Autism Speaks website has many helpful resources. The sleep toolkit (parent booklet) includes a discussion of many of the behavioral strategies discussed in this chapter. (The ATN/AIR-P materials are the product of ongoing activities of the Autism Speaks Autism Treatment Network, a program funded by Autism Speaks. It is supported by cooperative agreement UA3 MC 11054 through the U.S. Department of Health and Human Services, Health Resources and Services Administration, Maternal and Child Health Research Program to the Massachusetts General Hospital.)
- Durand, V.M. (1998). *Sleep Better! A Guide to Improving Sleep for Children with Special Needs.* Baltimore: Paul H. Brookes.
  This book describes sleep strategies for children with special needs.
- Ferber, R. (2006). *Solve Your Child's Sleep Problems.* 2nd ed. New York: Fireside.
  This book includes information about sleep basics, common sleep problems, and effective treatments.
- Friman, P. C. (2005). *Good Night, Sweet Dreams, I Love You; Now Get to Bed and Go to Sleep!* Boys Town, NE: Boys Town Press.
  This book provides general information about behavioral techniques, as well as specific sleep strategies including information about using a bedtime pass.
- Owens, J. A. and Mindell, J. (2005). *Take Charge of Your Child's Sleep: The All-in-One Resource for Solving Sleep Problems in Kids and Teens.* New York: Marlowe and Company.
  This is a review of common sleep problems and methods to address sleep difficulties in children and adolescents.

Other Resources

American Academy of Sleep Medicine (AASM)
One Westbrook Corporate Center, Suite 920
Westchester, IL 60154
708-492-0930; 708-492-0943 (fax)
www.aasmnet.org
www.sleepeducation.com

National Sleep Foundation (NSF)
1522 K Street, NW, Suite 500
Washington, DC 20005

202-341-3471; 202-341-3472 (fax)
www.sleepfoundation.org

Sleep Research Society (SRS)
One Westbrook Corporate Center, Suite 920
Westchester, IL 60154
708-492-0930; 708-492-0943 (fax)
www.sleepresearchsociety.org

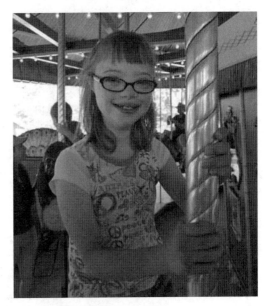

10

The Importance of Care Coordination for Children with DS-ASD

Cordelia Robinson, PhD, RN

Introduction

The purpose of this chapter is to offer families guidance as to how care coordination or case management can be a useful service and tool. Background information regarding the origins of the concept and how it has involved will be presented. The primary perspective that will be offered is what the definition, value, process, and outcomes of this service may mean for an individual with co-occurring Down syndrome and Autism Spectrum Disorder (DS-ASD) and his or her family. In addition, to help families to benefit fully from this service, this chapter will also address the role care coordination plays in our health care, social service, and educational systems.

Care Coordination versus Case Management

In this chapter, I will use the term care coordination. Another term that could reasonably be used is case management. In fact, the term case management is what you are likely to find in state and federal regulations. I believe the underlying functions to be accomplished are the same. I prefer to use the term care coordination for several reasons. The fundamental purpose of the work involves coordinating the efforts of everyone who is working with an individual and his or her family. An underlying assumption of coordination is the efficient and effective use of all resources. Resources are not just money to pay for services, but also the time and energy on the part of the individual with DS-ASD, his or her parents, and all the people who are part of development and implementation of the plan. Coordination requires clear and complete communication about all of the elements of the individual's daily experience across environments (Jackson, Finkler, & Robinson, 1992; 1995).

Another reason I prefer the term care coordination is because of the point of view articulated by families during the time the federal rules and regulations were being written for PL99-457 (the original early intervention law). The legislation used the term case management, presumably following from the term used in Medicaid regulations. However, families clearly said they did not like being thought of as "cases" nor did they wish to "be managed." Finally, I believe that the term "care" is a universal word that describes what all involved provide, whether the individual team member is the person, parent, family member, friend, or a paid provider from all disciplines. The work done to support the individual's and family's health, safety, well-being, and development is all done in the context of care giving.

Impact of Early Intervention Legislation on the Practice of Care Coordination

A major influence on the conceptualization of the role of care coordination came about with the passage of federal legislation. In 1986, federal legislation permitting states to receive federal funds to develop early intervention services for infants and toddlers (birth to three years) with developmental disabilities or developmental delays was passed. This legislation, PL99-457, became known as Part H and later, when the Education of the Handicapped Act was revised to become the Individuals with Disabilities Education Act (IDEA), it became known as Part C. In the early days of PL99-457, M.J. McGonigal, R.K. Kaufman, and B.H. Johnson (1991) offered this definition of Care Coordination:

> *"An active process for implementing intervention services that promote and support a family's capacities and competencies to identify, obtain, coordinate, monitor and evaluate resources and service to meet its needs" (p86).*

The context for this definition was the articulation of a family-centered approach, which was defined as an approach in which there is a respect for, and acceptance of, family diversity, promotion of the family as decision maker, and collaboration with professionals and programs that are responsible for family needs. This definition of case management (or care coordination) and the characteristics of family centered care had a major influence on the development of early intervention services under the federal legislation.

While there have been changes in the legislation over the years, a consistent mandate has been an entitlement to the services of service coordination for all eligible children with disabilities and their families. This service was to be provided at no expense to the family or to their insurance company. The inclusion of this service was driven at least in part by families who were receiving early intervention services, sometimes from many different providers. Families also reported receiving services from multiple service systems, such as health care and social services. Families reported that each of these service entities often appointed someone as "case manager." Parents complained that they needed to coordinate among the "case managers" as well as providers. It is presumably these observations from parents, and in some cases, providers, that laid the groundwork for the conceptualization of care coordination in PL99-457 and subsequent versions of the legislation.

The vision within the legislation was that a family should be able to have one person who could assist with coordination of all the services a family needed to support their child's development, health, and well-being. The legislation and the accompanying regulations anticipated one "case manager," with the selection based upon family preference and needs.

Another assumption underlying the legislation was that the federal funds would provide "glue money" that would permit transformation of systems so that a care coordinator would have authority to work across systems. The basis for this authority to work across systems was the fact that the legislation also mandated the development of an Individualized Family Service Plan (IFSP). The care coordinator in almost all states' early intervention systems is the person responsible for working with parents and providers to convene a meeting of all relevant parties to develop the IFSP and revise it at regular intervals. Again, the vision and the spirit of the legislation and regulations were well intended. However, actually convening a team at a time and location of the family's choosing was at times overwhelming, especially when team members came from multiple agencies. In my experience across several states, having the resources to bring an IFSP team together when different entities are paying for the different team members' work is extremely difficult.

Working with Your Early Intervention Care Coordinator

Early intervention legislation is fairly unique in the burden it places on the system to assist you in developing a comprehensive and functional plan for services to meet your child's developmental needs and to enhance your ability to meet your child's needs.

Open Communication: I believe you and your child's interests are best served when there is open communication among parents, care coordinators, and the child's providers. If your child's medical condition is complex and there are concerns about physical stamina, for example, bring that information to the IFSP meeting. If your child is in child care, your care coordinator should help you find a way for your care provider to receive information.

Individualized Services: Every provider should give you a rationale for what they are recommending for your child. They should be able to describe your child's current level of development and explain how their recommendations should enhance your child's development or day-to-day functioning. Providers should be able to tell you how they intend to document your child's progress and how they will change their plans based upon your child's progress or lack thereof. Neither you nor your care coordinator should accept a recommendation that just specifies a duration and frequency of a service (for example, physical therapy for thirty minutes, two times per week). Your child's IFSP should contain specific child behaviors as "outcomes" to be accomplished. If your child is receiving early intervention services in a specialized setting such as a hospital-based therapy department, be sure to ask for explanations as to how this intervention relates to your child's ability to engage in everyday play and routines at home.

Comprehensive Services: Early intervention services under the federal legislation are meant to be comprehensive. If the intervention you are receiving is not addressing activities of daily living such as self-feeding, toileting, dressing, and daily hygiene, and you need assistance with these areas, bring these issues up to your care coordinator so that they might be addressed in your child's IFSP. If your child's behavior is a problem, even if it seems as though it is perhaps just the "terrible twos," request consultation to assist you with this behavior. If you are worried about the adequacy of your child's diet or sleep, bring these issues up with your primary care provider for sure, but also with your care coordinator, since early intervention can assist with these issues. If your child would benefit from assistive technology, this issue should be addressed in the IFSP meeting.

Having a means of communication is an absolute priority. If your child is not using words to make her wants known, the possibility of using an alternative communication system should be discussed. In our study of the co-occurrence of DS-ASD (DiGiuseppi et al., 2010), we were very concerned about the number of children over four years of age who had no words, continued to receive traditional speech therapy, and were not given an alternative means of communication.

When we examine what services are provided under Part C, it tends to be almost exclusively physical, occupational, and speech and language therapies, and special instruction. However, there are many more services that are mandated including assistive tech services, health services, psychological services, and social work services, among others. It is incumbent upon your care coordinator and whatever agency employs him or her to assist you with these services.

Prioritizing Needs: I am not suggesting that getting everyone to an IFSP meeting and getting all of these issues addressed will be easy. There is a good chance that your Care Coordinator is assisting an additional 40 to 50 families. This reality of availability of time is not a trivial issue, so you may want to identify your own priorities where you need the most assistance. I strongly suggest that helping your child establish good sleep patterns, healthy eating habits, daily hygiene routines, and addressing any problem behaviors are as important as the traditional intervention issues of mobility and communication. In my experience, these activities of daily living are too often overlooked. However, these skills are extremely important to you and your child in both the short term and long term. Inclusion in school and neighborhood activities as well as family gatherings is facili-

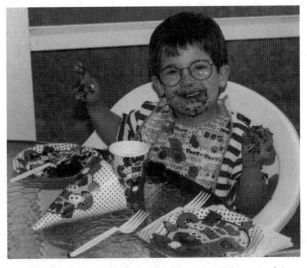

tated when your child with DS-ASD is able to be as independent as possible. Working on these skills may be difficult in the near term, but the payoff can be great. Don't feel as though you need to wait for your providers to bring up such issues. You have the right to request help in all domains of development and functioning.

The Primary Healthcare Provider's Role in Coordinating Your Child's Care

A definition of care coordination that reflects the importance of health care comes from a report by R.C. Antonelli, J.W. McAllister, and J. Popp (2009):

> *"Pediatric care coordination is a patient and family centered, assessment-driven, team based activity designed to meet the needs of children and youth while enhancing the care giving capabilities of families. Care Coordination addresses interrelated medical, social, developmental, behavioral, educational and financial needs in order to achieve optimal health and wellness outcomes."*

In the view of these writers, a critical related concept is that of Integrated Care. Integrated Care is defined as "the seamless and coordinated provision of health care services, from the perspective of the patient and family, across the entire care continuum, irrespective of institutional and departmental boundaries."

In other words, just as in the provision of early intervention services, there is a need to acknowledge and coordinate the interdependence of services from a variety of systems. All children benefit from having a regular source of health care. For children with DS-ASD, having access to primary care and specialist care is especially important. Over the past twenty years, as the concept and actual implementation of a medical home approach (Perrin et al., 2007) has become more commonplace, primary care providers have been playing a more active role in care coordination. For example, in the best circumstances, the Medical Home is fully informed and engaged about the services and supports their patients receive. With such information, the medical home is able to contribute any concerns and recommendations. A medical home should contribute a holistic perspective about an individual and her family.

Ideally, your child's early intervention and special education providers will consult with you and/or your child's medical providers when there are any concerns that health conditions could be affecting your child's development and learning. For example, sleep problems might be impairing your child's ability to learn new material.

Perhaps you have a service or care coordinator who works with you and your child in regards to early intervention or specialized therapy or educational service who does not ask about your child's health care. If this is the case, it is unfortunate. These two systems, health care and developmental and educational services, need to work together. If they are not in communication with one another, you should work to remedy that absence of communication. If your child receives care from mental healthcare providers, they need to be part of the communication system about your child's care as well. You should be sure to sign the paperwork to allow communication among all of these providers.

The concept of medical home, which was introduced and explicated by the American Academy of Pediatrics and the Maternal Child Health Bureau of the federal government, is meant to enable you and all providers for your child to have access to the critical information regarding your child's care. Don't think of your child's medical home as simply your child's primary healthcare provider. Rather, work with all of your child's providers so that there is a shared understanding of the concerns, priorities, and resources that are important to your child and your family. (See Chapter 6 for more information about the Medical Home concept.)

As a parent of a child with DS-ASD, you have come to understand the complex health and behavioral issues your child deals with. Down syndrome as a condition comes with a number of added health risks that you know to monitor and discuss with your child's primary care provider and specialists. Autism spectrum disorders come with many other problems as well.

It is too early in our awareness of the impact of co-occurrence of DS-ASD to know exactly how the risks of these two conditions interact. However, the combined health risks such as sleep disorders, nutritional problems, and risk for obesity, behavior and temperament issues, and anxiety disorders argue for ensuring that your child's primary care provider takes his or her role in care coordination seriously. It is essential that you have a primary care provider and specialty care providers who will work with you and your child to attend to not just acute health care concerns but to overall health and wellness concerns. Developmental progress is important, but overall health and wellness are a critical aspect of daily life for you and your child with DS-ASD (Robinson, 2009).

Colorado Care Coordination Community of Practice

The emphasis placed on care coordination in Medicaid waivers, early intervention (Part C), and the medical home highlight the critical need for communication and coordination across service systems if individuals, their families, and society as a whole are to receive maximum benefit from investments made in services and supports. This is true whether these investments are made from individual and family resources or public resources (McDonald et al., 2011).

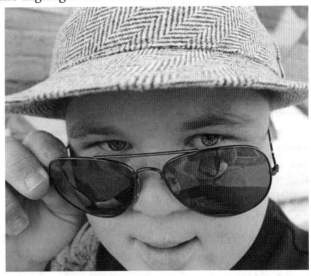

In response to the point that many agencies provide care coordination, frequently to some of the same people, a number of people in Colorado came together in an effort to articulate a common definition of care coordination to be used across agencies and groups of individuals in Colorado. The work of developing a definition and toolkit began under a federal grant, Project Bloom (Colorado Department of Human Services and JFK Partners, University of Colorado School of Medicine), and its continued development has evolved to include collaboration with the Colorado Department of Public Health and Environment. The underlying premise of the work was the fact that families still encounter many care coordinators, depending upon the complexity of their needs. With these multiple coordinators come multiple plans for their children and themselves. Each of these plans and coordinators are governed by multiple and different regulations, creating potential difficulties for families and potential inefficiencies in use of resources. From long experience with systems, we did not expect agencies and systems to give up their regulations and forms. We decided instead to see if we could get all the different players to agree upon the functions to be served with care coordination across all agencies and populations.

This group self identifies as the Colorado Care Coordination Community of Practice (CCCCP). As a Community of Practice, we are talking to every group we can to give us an audience. We ask for their input to refine the statements. We ask that they envision health, mental health, social service, and educational systems that agree on the functions outlined here as the expectations for their work with individuals and families. We ask that they envision systems that set an expectation that their personnel reach out, with family permission, to their counterparts in other agencies. The definition of care coordination developed by this community of practice is:

Table 10-1: Colorado Care Coordination Community of Practice, Values, and Functions

Values of Care Coordination

The values underlying the provision of care coordination services are as follows:
- To provide a team-based, partnership approach;
- To make a commitment to provide family-centered care;
- To build on the strengths of the family and to work with the family in developing the plan;
- To share pertinent and appropriate information across systems (among all providers and the family);
- To provide accurate information that is understandable to everyone involved in the individual's and his or her family's plan;
- To utilize culturally responsive practices;
- To recognize that families have different levels and types of care coordination needs;
- To match the type and timing of care coordination to the family's needs;
- To recognize that parents are the continuity between, and have the authority of managing, the services and supports they receive;
- To involve the family in contributing to the description of specific activities;
- To be available and accessible as needed over time.

Functions of Care Coordination

- Assess with the family and individual their strengths as well as unmet needs across life domains;
- Identify all sources of referrals, services, and supports, facilitate connections with these sources, and manage continuous communication across these sources;
- Identify desired outcomes for the individual and his or her family;
- Develop a comprehensive plan of care and services with the family or individual that includes a plan to address unmet needs;
- Provide information around the purpose and function of recommended referrals, services, and supports;
- Periodically and as needed reassess and modify the plan of care with the individual and his or her family;
- Support and facilitate transitions, including transitions in and out of care coordination;
- Clearly identify responsibilities for each party to the plan;
- Share knowledge and information across systems, and facilitate communication, among all parties of the plan.

> *Care coordination addresses interrelated medical, social, developmental, behavioral, educational, and financial needs to optimize health and wellness outcomes. Care coordination is a person-and family-centered, assessment-driven, team activity designed to meet the needs and preferences of individuals while enhancing the care giving capabilities of families and service providers.*

The Values and Functions developed by the CCCCP are presented here in Table 10-1 on page 136 as a framework to provide a comprehensive view of care coordination. In Table 10-2 below we identify outcomes of care coordination that we expect to see at both individual and system levels.

There is a toolkit that expands upon the definition, values, functions and outcomes available at http://jfkpartners.org/default.asp?page=12. We encourage families to take a look at this material and assess their current needs, priorities, and expectations from any public systems they may interact with. While it is reasonable to have expectations for assistance from these systems and the assistance of a care coordinator, a self-appraisal of areas of concern is probably a good starting point for you as an individual family.

A commonality among the definitions of care coordination offered here is that they present an ideal view. The families who met with us and contributed to the definitions and toolkit almost universally indicated that they were the primary care coordinator for their family member. Some were at points in their lives where they accepted this reality and others were angry about the difficulties in coordination. All of them desired a better situation and contributed to what you see here.

As a parent of a child who has two complex disorders that affect his or her health and development, you are going to learn and become the expert in many aspects of your child's care. One of the challenges you face is that of not permitting these two conditions (Down syndrome and autism) to define your child and your family. Care coordination and the services that care coordination seeks to organize can be useful to accomplishing your goals, but hopefully do not come to define the fabric of your daily life.

Table 10-2: Colorado Care Coordination Community of Practice Outcomes

Well-being and Satisfaction:
- Family/individual goals achieved;
- Reduction in percentage of unmet needs;
- Increase family/individual satisfaction;
- Increase provider satisfaction;
- Family functioning is healthy/improved;
- Family feels knowledgeable.

(continued on next page)

(continued from previous page)

Process:
- Ease of access to resource information;
  - Increased individual/family and provider access to information about available resources;
  - Increased positive individual/family "teach-back" skills demonstrated;
- Enhanced communication among providers/family/community partners;
  - Increased documentation of care plan use and oversight;
- Single point of entry into multiple services/single coordination function across multiple services.

Community and Relationship Supports:
- Improved relationships with family and friends;
- Improved parent-child relationships;
- Positive social supports;
  - Access to community resources including: Recreation, Transportation, Spiritual, Legal, Education.

Functional Essentials:
- Increased self-management skills;
- Increased functional abilities;
  - Increased functional assessment, school attendance/success, ability to perform activities of daily living;
- Support achievement of developmental trajectory;
  - Functional levels achieved, milestones marked;
- Basic needs and essentials are met that include the following: Income, Home, Utilities, Food, Clothing, Insurance, Transportation, Childcare.

Physical and Mental Health and Development:
- Enhance communication between family and all sources of service and support;
  - Reduce percentage of children seen by specialist without information from PCP; reduced percentage of children seen by PCP without information from consultation/specialist;
- Increased measures of health;
  - Health goals reached, family perception of individual's health increased;
- Increase activity, developmental screening, and health promotion (Early and Periodic Screening, Diagnosis, and Treatment Guidelines, AAP and Bright Futures Guidelines);
  - Increased percentage of all children screened for developmental delays and sensory deficits by select periodic well-child visits and/or school entry;
- Improve access to health and mental health care.

References

Antonelli, R.C., McAllister, J.W., & Popp, J. (May 2009). Making care coordination a critical component of the pediatric health system: A multidisciplinary framework. *The Commonwealth Fund.*

Bailey, D. (1989). Case management in early intervention. *Journal of Early Intervention 13(2):*120-34.

DiGuiseppi, C., Hepburn, S., Davis, J.M., Fidler, D.J., Hartway, S., Raitano, L., Miller, L., Ruttenberg, M., & Robinson, C. (2010). Screening for autism spectrum disorders in children with Down syndrome: Population prevalence and screening test characteristics. *Journal of Developmental Behavioral Pediatrics 31(3):* 181-91.

Jackson, B., Finkler, D., & Robinson, C. (1992). A case management system for infants with chronic illnesses and developmental disabilities. *Children's Health Care 21(4):* 224-31.

Jackson, B., Finkler, D., & Robinson, C. (1995). A cost analysis of a case management system for infants with chronic illness and developmental disease. *Journal of Pediatric Nursing 10(5):* 304-10.

JFK Partners Care Coordination. http://jfkpartners.org/default.asp?page=106

McDonald, K.M., Schultz, E., Albin, L., Pineda, N., Lonhart, J., Sundaram, V., Smith-Spangler, C., Brustrom, J., & Malcolm, E. (January 2011). *Care Coordination Measures Atlas.* (AHRQ Publication No. 11-0023-EF). Rockville, MD: Agency for Healthcare Research and Quality. http://www.ahrq.gov/qual/careatlas/.

McGonigal, M.J., Kaufmann, R.K., & Johnson, B.H. (1991). *Guidelines and Recommended Practices for the Individualized Family Service Plan.* 2nd ed. Bethesda, MD: Association for the Care of Children's Health.

Perrin, J.M., Romm, D., Bloom, S.R., Homer, C.J., Kuhlthau, K.A., Cooley, C., Duncan, P., Roberts, R., Slayer, P., Wells, N., & Newacheck, P. (2007). A family-centered, community-based system for services for children and youth with special health care needs. *Archives of Pediatric and Adolescent Medicine 161(10):* 933-36.

Robinson, C. (2009). What nurses need to know about the other ASD. *Journal for Specialists in Pediatric Nursing 14(3):* 155-56.

Singer, S.J., Burgers, J., Friedberg, M., Rosenthal, M.B., Leape, L., & Schneider, E. (2011). Defining and measuring integrated patient care: Promoting the next frontier in health care delivery. *Medical Care Research and Review (68)1:* 112-27

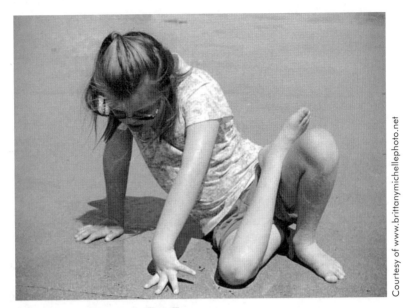

Courtesy of www.brittanymichellephoto.net

11

Addressing Problem Behaviors in Individuals with DS-ASD

Sam Towers, MA

Why Problem Behavior Is Used

Behavior is purposeful, meaning that people use behavior to achieve goals that are important to them. This is true of all people, whether they have DS-ASD or not. People use specific behaviors because those behaviors previously have helped them to achieve what they want, or they have observed another person use the behavior successfully to achieve what he wants.

As such, behavior can be viewed as a form of communication, regardless of whether the individual using the behavior intends to use it as communication. In other words, we can "read" an individual's behavior to learn what that individual is attempting to achieve through the use of the behavior.

For example, if a child hits his mother in an attempt to get an apple, the child could be viewed as saying something like, "Mom, I want an apple, and you'd better figure out quickly that I want an apple, or I am going to keep hitting you." Although these may not be the thoughts that are going through the child's mind, the child knows that hitting his mother has resulted, at least occasionally, in getting what he wants.

Problem behavior often is the result of a skill deficit, meaning that the individual using it does not have the appropriate skills to achieve what he wants to achieve. In the example above, the child might not have the ability to communicate that he wants an apple. In these cases, the individual should be taught the skills necessary to achieve the goals that are important to him.

At times, an individual might use problem behavior even if he has the appropriate skills because the problem behavior pays off for him more quickly and/or more consistently. In the example above, the child might have been able to ask for an apple by saying "apple." Instead he knew that he would be more likely to get the apple if he hit his mother while pointing to the apple because sometimes when asked for an apple, she did not give it to him. Or perhaps he had learned that he would get the apple more quickly if he hit her because when he hasn't hit her, she has taken longer to get an apple for him.

Whatever the case, it is highly likely that the individual is using this behavior because it has paid off previously. It has helped him to get something before. He has learned from the consequences of the behavior.

Improving Behavior

Rapport

It is important that everyone who works with an individual with DS-ASD build rapport with him. Rapport is a positive relationship between two or more people. The foundation of all interventions is well-built rapport. Those who have well-built rapport will be much more able to prevent an individual with DS-ASD from using problem behavior and will be much more able to provide support when an individual with DS-ASD uses problem behavior. In addition, and perhaps most importantly, the more people with whom an individual with DS-ASD has well-built rapport, the richer his life will be.

To develop rapport with an individual with DS-ASD, or anyone for that matter, do the following:

- *Frequently engage the individual in a wide variety of activities that he finds enjoyable.* Relationships are built upon people having fun together.

   Ensure that there is at least an 8:1 ratio of positive interactions to negative interactions. Praise and compliments are examples of positive interactions. Corrective feedback (e.g., "You missed a spot") is an example of a negative interaction. People typically like positive people. One way to ensure you engage in many more positive interactions than negative interactions is to "catch the individual being good." Catching an individual being good is intentionally looking for things the individual is doing well and praising the individual for it.

At times, during the busyness of our lives, it is hard to remember to catch an individual doing good. One way to remember is to put a large number of marbles or other objects in one of your pockets. There should be enough marbles so that you will notice them frequently. When you notice the marbles, look to see if the individual is being good. If so, praise the individual and then take a marble out of your pocket and put it into another pocket.

Transferring the marbles to another pocket will help you keep track of how many times you have caught the individual being good. If you get all the marbles into the other pocket, then start putting them back into the first pocket. It is very helpful if you set a goal each day for how many marbles you will move from one pocket to another. By the time you get used to having the marbles in your pocket and don't notice them anymore, you probably will be in the habit of catching the individual being good.

- **Ensure that you engage in many more non-demand interactions than demand interactions.** Demand interactions are interactions in which you are asking the individual to do something (e.g., "Please look at me"). Non-demand interactions are interactions in which you do not ask the individual to do something (e.g., "Hi, it is good to see you").

Imagine that you know that, every time you see a particular neighbor coming, the neighbor is going to ask to borrow something. The neighbor never comes to visit, to give help, or to do anything except ask for something. Soon, when you see that neighbor coming, you might look for a closet to hide in. Individuals with DS-ASD might not be able to find a place to hide, but they certainly can build "walls" that will keep people who only make demands on them from having a meaningful relationship with them.

It is often best not to make any requests when first building rapport. As time goes on, you can start introducing requests; however, these initial requests should be ones with which the individual can easily comply.

- **Provide the individual with many, many successful experiences.** Helping him to achieve success will help him to see you in a positive light.
- **Be genuine in all your interactions with the individual.** If you are insincere with him, it may impede your relationship with him.
- **Interact with the individual in a kind and caring manner.** Do not be harsh with him. There will be times that it will be fine to be firm, but harshness will damage rapport.
- **Do not interact with the individual in a condescending manner.** Some people with DS-ASD understand what condescension is, and they would like to be treated as an equal.

At times, the rapport building process can't start until the individual feels comfortable with the person who is attempting to build rapport. Some individuals with DS-ASD can be very apprehensive of new people. If so, they will not be ready for the procedures above. In these cases, begin by just being around the individual without interacting with him or getting too close to him. For example, you could go to the individual's classroom, talk with the teacher, and help other students. Over time, the individual with DS-ASD should become more comfortable with you. At that point, you should interact for brief periods of time with him in activities that he enjoys (e.g., give him his snacks at snack time). Once the individual becomes more comfortable with you, you can increase the amount of time spent with him and use the procedures above.

Don't Let Problem Behavior Be Successful

People use behavior to achieve goals that are important to them. When a behavior results in an individual achieving a goal, that behavior has been successful; it has paid off. For example, a girl might use self-biting in an attempt to escape a task (e.g., participating in a skill-building session). If she is allowed to escape the task, the behavior has been successful for her; it has paid off.

It is important not to let problem behavior be successful. If a problem behavior pays off, the individual is likely to use the behavior again and again in an attempt to achieve the same goals and perhaps to achieve other goals. If a behavior does not pay off, over time the individual will use the behavior less and less.

For example, if someone with DS-ASD yells and screams in an attempt to get your attention, you should not provide attention. Please note that the following are all forms of attention: (a) talking to him; (b) making eye contact with him: (c) being in close proximity to him; (d) making physical contact with him; (e) talking about him in his presence; and (f) saying his name in his presence.

It is important to note that if a child tantrums while in public (e.g., in a grocery store), it is fine to leave the setting immediately. If you have to leave something behind, such as a grocery cart with groceries, there are people who are paid to put the stuff back where it belongs.

When not allowing the behavior to be successful, you should be aware of the possibility of an **extinction burst.** An extinction burst is an escalation in problem behavior that occurs if the problem behavior is no longer successful. For example, let's say that screaming has worked for your child to get milk, and you have decided that you are no longer going to give the him milk when he screams. At first, the screaming will get worse. It may get louder. It may last longer. Your child might even throw in another problem behavior with it.

Extinction bursts occur because the behavior has paid off for the individual before, but it isn't paying off now. An individual's thought processes might go something like this. "This used to work. I must be doing something wrong. Maybe I am not loud enough. Maybe I need to do it longer. I know this used to work, and I bet I can get it to work again if I only try hard enough." The individual's actual thought processes might not be working in quite this manner, but, in any event, his behavior will likely escalate in an attempt to get the behavior to be successful again.

The Importance of Consistency: The key here is not to give in. If you give in, you have just taught the individual that escalating his problem behavior works. So, if you stop allowing a behavior to be successful, be consistent and don't give in. If you consistently don't give in, the behavior will finally decrease to much lower levels.

Consistency is very important for another reason. If you are inconsistent and give in occasionally, you likely will teach the individual to keep trying the behavior because it pays off sometimes. The following is a story that illustrates this.

In this story, I use a blender every morning to make a fruit smoothie for breakfast. The behavior in this example is pushing the button on the blender. The payoff is the blender blending my smoothie. The blender is nine years old. One morning, after I put everything in the blender, I push the button, and the blender doesn't work. I check and see that it is plugged in. I push the button again, and the blender works. I briefly wonder why it didn't work the first time, but soon my thoughts are occupied with other things.

The next morning when I push the button, the blender doesn't work. Again I check and see that it is plugged in. I push the button again, and again the blender doesn't work. I push the button again, but with force this time. (Ah, an extinction burst!) Again the blender doesn't work. I push the button two more times before it works, and I am beginning to think that it might be time for a new blender.

The next morning I push the button, and again the blender doesn't work. In fact, I have to push the button twelve times to get it to work. I am now convinced that I should get a new blender, but I forget to buy one.

The next morning, I look at the blender and wish that I had remembered to buy a new blender. I push the button once, and the blender works! I am now thinking that the blender may have fixed itself. (Yeah, right.)

The next morning, I have to push the button twenty-seven times before it works. I make a note to buy a new blender that evening, but again, I forget.

The next morning, the blender works on the fifth push of the button, and I wonder, "What's up with this crazy blender?"

The next morning, I push the button fifty times, and it never does work. I take everything out of the blender, I throw the blender away, and I buy a new one that night.

Let's examine this story. If I would have had to push the button fifty times to get it to work when it first started to fail, I would not have pushed the button fifty times. I would have given up long before. So why did I push the button fifty times on that last morning? I pushed it fifty times because that mindless little machine had taught to me to think, "Maybe it will work this time." It had taught me to think, "Maybe this time," because it had worked sometimes, and it had worked in such an unpredictable manner (e.g., the fifth time, the twelfth time, the first time, the twenty-seventh time), that I never knew for sure when it would work.

The gambling industry makes a lot of money using the principle of behavior. Slot machines don't pay off every time, but they pay off just often enough to make people think, "Maybe this time."

The same thing happens with the behavior of individuals with DS-ASD. If a behavior has paid off only some of the time, the individual will use it for a much longer period time even if it stops paying off all together.

There are two lessons here. The first is not to give in during an extinction burst because the individual will learn to escalate his behavior in order to get it to pay off. The second lesson is that, when you decide not to allow a behavior to pay off any more, make sure you are consistent in not allowing a payoff, or it will take much longer to decrease, or perhaps it never will decrease.

In the Event of an Emergency: There are some situations in which it will not be possible to keep the behavior from providing some payoff to the individual. In these situations, ensure that the behavior has the least amount of payoff possible. For example, if your child sits in the middle of a street in an attempt to get attention, in most instances you will have to move him. That means that you will have to provide some attention (e.g., coming into close proximity and making physical contact). If this occurs, minimize the amount of other types of attention you provide. Do not speak to your child unless necessary, do not make eye contact unless necessary, and do not speak about your child. So, even though the behavior has paid off somewhat, it hasn't paid off as much as your child probably wanted.

Please note that it is very difficult, if not impossible, for anyone to be completely consistent. With that said, be as consistent as you can be, and don't beat yourself up if you aren't 100 percent consistent. If you are inconsistent, just make a plan to keep that inconsistency from happening again.

The Rewards of Consistency: In the end, at times, the ride can be pretty rough when you decide not to allow a behavior to be successful; however, you can comfort yourself with these two thoughts. The first is that if you remain consistent, things will finally get better. The second and more important thought is that you are helping the individual to lead a better and richer life.

New Experiences

Many people with DS-ASD experience a lot of anxiety/fear about new experiences. This can include going to new places, meeting new people, engaging in new activities, eating new foods, and watching new movies. People with DS-ASD like their world to be very predictable, and new experiences are often not predictable for them.

Imagine yourself being plopped down in a totally unfamiliar country. The language is different. The customs are different. Social expectations are different. Everything is different. For many people this would be a very unsettling experience, perhaps even a frightening one.

Over time, you might come to learn some of the language, and you might figure out what is expected socially in a few situations, but more often than not, just as you think you have figured out what is expected in another social situation, the expectations seem to change radically and for no apparent reason.

Then the people you live with bring you to a large event with a lot of new people and new experiences. Nothing seems to make sense. The sounds are very loud, and the lights are too bright. It seems like every ten to fifteen seconds, something unexpected and startling is happening. It seems that you can't do anything right. People are upset with you. Some of them even yell at you. Soon you feel like you want to cry, and you really want to go home, where, although things aren't fully comfortable, at least you usually know what is going to happen.

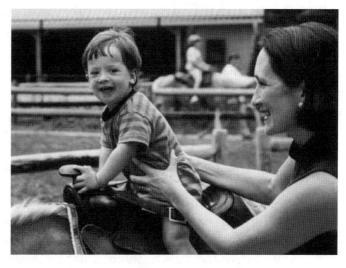

After situations like this happen to you a few times, you don't want to go anywhere new, meet anyone new, or do anything new. The world is already too crazy to have to try to deal with something new.

People with DS-ASD might be living a life somewhat like this. Two things should be done to help people with DS-ASD with new situations. One is to expose them to a new situation gradually. The other is to teach them skills to handle new situations well.

Priming

Priming is one way to help people with DS-ASD become accustomed to a new situation gradually. Priming is letting the individual have a sneak preview of the new situation. For example, if parents know that their child will be going on a field trip to a museum next week, they could take the child to the museum on the weekend and do a quick tour through the museum. It will not be necessary to take a lengthy tour and talk a lot about what they see in the museum. All they should be trying to accomplish is to help the child become familiar with the museum so that when he returns with his class, he will be somewhat familiar with the museum.

Priming can also be used to introduce new academic concepts or activities of daily living to an individual with DS-ASD. For example, if a child is having difficulty attending during story time at school, one evening the parents can read the next day's story to the child. This can help the child to become more familiar with the story, which could result in the child having greater interest in the story the next day.

Social Stories

Social Stories are another way to help individuals become accustomed to a new situation. Social Stories, a la Carol Gray, can be used to describe a new situation prior to the individual being exposed to the situation. Often, knowing about a new situation before encountering it helps individuals with DS-ASD to feel more comfortable with the situation once in it. Social Stories can be used to help the individual to:

- Understand what is going to occur in a situation.
- Know what things might look like in the new situation.
- Know who might be there.
- Understand the perspective of others in the situation, such as what other people might think, feel, and believe. Knowing this information can be used to help the individual understand other people's motivations for acting the way they do. It can also help an individual with DS-ASD to understand how others in the situation might respond to the behaviors that the individual with DS-ASD might use.
- Understand what is expected in that situation.
- Understand how to respond appropriately in the situation. This information is very important, because not only should the individual with DS-ASD know what is happening in the situation and why it is happening, but he should also learn the skills necessary to be socially successful in the situation. A social story can help him do just that.

Social Stories frequently have comprehension questions at the end. These questions help to ensure that the individual understands the story. In addition, role-playing often is used after a story to help the individual practice the skills that he will be using in the situation.

The use of visual representations (e.g., pictures, line drawings, and icons) in Social Stories can be very helpful because they will allow the individual to become a little more familiar with the situation prior to actually being in the situation.

A very good book explaining how to teach Social Stories is *The New Social Stories Book: Illustrated Edition,* written by Carol Gray (see Suggested Reading). The book contains many pre-written Social Stories for common situations; however, instructions are provided for writing Social Stories for situations that are not covered in the book.

Escape Motivated Behaviors

At times, people with DS-ASD will use problem behavior to escape tasks that they don't like. In these situations, if the individual is capable of performing the task, ensure that he does not escape the task. If you allow him to escape the task, he will likely use problem behavior again when asked to perform that task and perhaps even when asked to do others. One way to accomplish this is to deny the individual access to preferred objects and activities until he completes the task. For example, you might not allow the individual to do anything else fun until the task is done.

At times, it might be best not to ask the individual to complete the entire task. For example, if he appears to be unduly stressed by the task, you might ask him to complete only the next step or two of the task and not require him to complete the entire task. You should only ask someone not to complete the entire task when you believe that, for whatever reason, he does not have the ability to complete the entire task.

After an individual has used problem behavior in an attempt to avoid a task, try to determine why he did not comply, and, if appropriate, make modifications or accommodations. Some reasons that might have interfered with an individual's ability to complete the task are:

- The individual was not capable of performing the task because he did not have the prerequisite skills for performing the task. In this case, make sure that the individual has the prerequisite skills. For example, if the individual was asked to button his shirt, but did not have the prerequisite fine motor skills to do so, he should not be asked to button a shirt again until he has developed the fine motor skills necessary for buttoning his shirt.
- The task appeared too big to him to complete in one sitting. In these cases, the task can be broken down into smaller units.
- Something occurred that made it difficult for the individual to complete the task. For example, the environment was too noisy, the individual had a poor night's sleep the night before, or he was hungry. In these cases, work to mitigate the problem(s). For example, give your child something to eat if he is hungry.

Transitions

A significant number of individuals with DS-ASD have difficulty successfully navigating transitions, often resulting in the use of problem behavior. Some of the transitions that can be difficult are transitioning from working with one person to working with another, transitioning from one activity to another, and transitioning from one location to another. At times, individuals with DS-ASD are expected to make all three of those transitions at the same time.

Unexpected transitions can be especially difficult. Too many people with DS-ASD don't know what will be happening next. To one degree or another, most people feel more comfortable when they know what will be happening in their lives. To help people with DS-ASD know what is coming next, we can use routines and schedules.

An individual with DS-ASD should have a relatively consistent routine throughout the day. This predictability in his day will help him to anticipate the upcoming transitions and be better prepared to navigate them. This routine should not be rigid. In other words, the routine should change some from day to day. A routine that is rigid and inflexible can leave an individual with DS-ASD rigid and inflexible, leading to a much poorer quality of life.

Visual schedules often can be very useful for helping an individual to navigate transitions successfully. A visual schedule is a set of pictures, icons, written words, and/or objects that communicate a series of activities or the steps of a specific activity. Ideally, they communicate clear expectations to the individual and decrease the need for support.

To help an individual navigate a transition, give the individual prior notice of a transition. This prior notice should include an explanation of the transition (e.g., what the next activity will be and what will be occurring in it) and how long it will be until the transition occurs. The length of time until the transition occurs should be made as explicit to him as possible. One way to make the length of time more explicit is to tell him what will occur prior to the transition. For example, you might say, "When the show is over, it will be time to take a shower."

Another way to make the length of time more explicit is to use a visual timer. A visual timer displays a visual representation of remaining time in a more concrete manner than standard clocks or timers. For example, one type of visual timer is a small tower with three sections. The bottom section is green, the middle section is yellow, and the top section is red. This timer can be set up to have the green section lit for the first 80 percent of the desired time. At the end of that period of time, the green section flashes, turns off, and the yellow section is lit for 15 percent of the time. At the end of that time, the yellow section flashes, turns off, and the red section is lit for the remaining 5 percent of the time. Finally, the red section flashes, turns off, and the timer says something like, "Time's up."

If there is an unanticipated change in the individual's schedule or routine, he should be provided with as much advance notice as possible. He should be told of the change, when it will occur, and why it will occur. If he is using a visual schedule, the visual schedule should be changed to reflect the change in schedule.

Please note that, in my experience, the vast majority of individuals with disabilities do better when provided with a schedule of upcoming activities. However, some individuals actually do worse if they know what activities will be occurring. In some cases, the individual might become very anxious when told that a change in his routine will be occurring later. At times, that anxiety can lead to problem behavior. In some cases, an individual might become overly excited when told that a highly preferred activity will be occurring later in the day. He might become so excited that it will be difficult for him to complete the activities before that activity. In these instances, it might be best if the individual is not told of activities until shortly before they occur. Even more importantly, the individual should be taught self-calming skills so that he can anticipate activities in his schedule without encountering too much difficulty.

Examples of calming skills that help some individuals include:

- Using self-talk, such as telling oneself something like, "Everything will be okay. I've been able to do this before."
- Listening to music that has a calming effect on the individual.
- Progressive muscle relaxation.
- Engaging in identified sensory-based calming activities, such as swinging, deep pressure, or jumping on a trampoline.

At times, a person with DS-ASD might have difficulty with a transition because he is being asked to transition from a more preferred activity to a less preferred activity. In these cases, remind him of other pleasant activities on his schedule that will be available once he navigates the transition. For example, if he is having difficulty transitioning from watching a video to doing a chore, remind him that the next thing on his schedule after the chore is a ride to the park. Please note that you should not offer something that is not already on the schedule. For example, if a ride to the park is not the next thing on the schedule after the chore, don't offer him a ride to the park if he does the chore. If you do so, he might learn that he will get something fun if he refuses a transition. This will then encourage him to refuse transitions.

Individuals with DS-ASD would likely be served well by having some major changes in their lives introduced gradually. For example, if an adult with DS-ASD needs to move into a new home, it likely would be best to have him visit the new home and interact with the people in this home many times prior to moving into the new home.

Self-Stimulatory Behaviors

Many people with DS-ASD use self-stimulatory behaviors, and some of them use these behaviors quite frequently. Self-stimulatory behaviors are behaviors that are used only for the sensation(s) that the individual gets from the behavior. Some examples of self-stimulatory behaviors are:

- watching a fan turn;
- repeatedly flushing a toilet to watch the water go down;
- self-slapping;
- repeatedly flicking a string in front of the eyes; and
- making sounds just for the enjoyment of hearing the sounds or the feeling of the vibrations when sounds are made.

Self-stimulatory behaviors are not used to get a payoff from other people. One of the hallmarks of self-stimulatory behaviors is that they are used, at least some of the time, when the person is alone. No one else has to be present; the self-stimulatory behaviors carry their own payoff. All people use some self-stimulatory behaviors. Some people listen to music for the pure enjoyment of hearing the music. Some eat chocolate for the pure enjoyment of the flavor of chocolate. Some twirl their hair, and might not even recognize that they are doing it.

In and of themselves, self-stimulatory behaviors are not a problem; however, they can become a problem in the following situations:

- When the behaviors interfere with being more fully included in social interactions. For example, some people avoid others who are using self-stimulatory behaviors and/or say things like, "Watch out for that guy. He does some really weird stuff."

- Although people who provide support to individuals who use self-stimulatory behaviors might not be bothered much by these behaviors, many other people are bothered by them and sometimes even fearful of people who use certain self-stimulatory behaviors.
- When the behaviors consume so much of the individual's time that he does not have adequate time to learn important skills.
- When the behaviors consume so much time that the individual engages in few other activities. Essentially, it can result in the individual living in "his own world." This can severely limit the number of things that the individual can learn to enjoy, including social interactions.

Increasing An Individual's Range of Interests

It is thought that individuals with DS-ASD use self-stimulatory behaviors, at least in part, because they haven't learned to enjoy other activities. In other words, they have a limited range of interests. If so, one way to decrease self-stimulatory behaviors is to increase the individual's range of interests. In addition to helping decrease self-stimulatory behaviors, it is important for an individual to have an ever-growing number of interests for the following reasons:

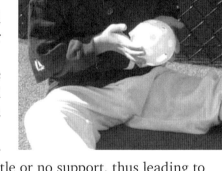

- He will lead a richer life because he has more things to enjoy.
- An increased range of interests will lead to increased opportunities for him to interact with others.
- These new interests might become very fun for the individual, and could be used to reward him when learning new skills.
- These new interests might be activities that he can accomplish with little or no support, thus leading to greater independence and a decreased need for support from others.

The following are some considerations and procedures for introducing an individual to new interests:

- Some individuals with DS-ASD are reluctant to try new activities because they don't know what to expect from new things. If so, introduce the interest gradually, so as to allow the person to become comfortable with and know what to expect from it.
- Don't give up if he initially rejects a new activity. It may be that he has not become comfortable enough with the new interest to determine

whether he likes it or not. Provide him with enough exposures so that he can determine whether or not he truly dislikes the new interest. Please note that you should not force him to participate in the new interest. Instead, slowly expose him to the new interest. I have seen a number of individuals, both with and without disabilities, who initially did not prefer a new activity, but came to enjoy it greatly after repeated exposures.

- Make the new activity/item seem fun and inviting to him. For example, speak about it in an exciting manner either when first introducing it to him or when exposing him to it indirectly.
- Reward him for participating in new activities. This reward will help to encourage him to participate in the new activities until he can determine if he likes them.
- Expose him to new interests that have characteristics of current interests. For example, if the individual enjoys swimming, you might try developing his interest in other water activities. Or if he greatly likes the color red, you could buy him red toys.
- In addition, you can use the procedures in the section above titled "New Experiences" to help an individual become accustomed to potential new interests.

It is important to note that nobody enjoys everything to which he is introduced. After all, there are people in this world who do not enjoy hot, spicy food even after being introduced to it many times. The key is to make sure that the individual has had adequate opportunities to experience a new interest so he can make an informed decision as to whether or not he likes the new interest.

Self-Stimulatory Behaviors Used for Self-Soothing

It is also thought that some individuals who use self-stimulatory behaviors use these behaviors, at least in part, to soothe themselves. We should not deprive an individual with DS-ASD from self-soothing, but if the self-soothing behavior results in the individual being excluded socially or otherwise restricting his ability to enjoy life to the fullest, alternative methods of self-soothing should be explored with the individual. For example, a child could be taught to listen to calming music through headphones, if he can tolerate headphones, or he could be taught to provide himself with deep pressure in an unobtrusive manner. The individual can be taught to use the more appropriate soothing skill using the procedures in the section below that is titled "Teaching a Replacement Behavior."

Setting Events Can Complicate Things

Certain events in a person's life can change the way that the person typically behaves. These events are called setting events, and many of them can be thought of as changing a person's mood. Negative setting events can worsen a person's mood. Positive setting events can improve a person's mood.

The following are some setting events that can be negative for some people with DS-ASD:

- change in routine;
- being sick;
- being tired;
- having been involved in conflict;
- being told of something disappointing;
- being under the care of someone new;
- lack of familiarity with people in a setting;
- boredom;
- moving to a new home, new school, etc.;
- noisy environments;
- crowded environments;
- environments with a lot of commotion;
- pain;
- hunger;
- lighting; and
- temperature.

This list could go on and on.

Positive setting events are things that a person enjoys. The following are some setting events that can be positive for people with DS-ASD, depending upon whether they enjoy them:

- praise;
- one-on-one attention;
- eating preferred foods; and
- engaging in preferred activities.

Again this list could go on and on.

There are tools we can use when someone is experiencing the effects of a negative setting event. The first tool is to *get rid of or minimize the setting event.* For example, if we find out that the individual is in pain, we should take steps to alleviate the pain (e.g., give a mild pain reliever, or take the individual to a doctor). Or if the individual is sleeping poorly because of the noisy college students who just moved in next door, perhaps we can put sound insulation in the bedroom window and provide some white noise to cover the neighbors' sounds. Perhaps we could move the person to a bedroom on the other side of the house.

Another tool is to *use positive setting events to help offset some of the effects of negative setting events.* The following is an example of how to use positive setting events to offset the effect of negative setting events. If a child with DS-ASD has had a poor night's sleep and he is missing his father who has been away for three days on business, the school could do one or more of the following to help increase the likelihood that the child will have a better day.

- A preferred person could provide the child with a lot of praise and attention when he first arrives at school. For some children with DS-ASD, praise and attention from a preferred person can help improve their moods.
- The child could be given increased one-on-one attention throughout the day. Again, for some children with DS-ASD, this can help to improve their moods.
- His schedule could be modified so that he has more fun activities throughout the day than is usual.
- More choice in his schedule could be provided. Choice can be a strong tool to help increase motivation.

A third tool that can minimize the effect of negative setting events is to *decrease the challenges that an individual experiences.* When an individual is experiencing the effects of a negative setting event, he might not have his usual capacity for dealing with challenges. For example, in the above situation, the following could be done:

- The academic demands could be decreased somewhat.
- Any exceptionally challenging activities could be avoided completely. For example, asking a child experiencing the effects of negative setting events to take a long ride on a crowded and noisy bus for a field trip can be asking for disaster.

There are considerations for using these procedures. They are:

- Use these procedures *before* the individual with DS-ASD starts using a problem behavior. Providing a positive setting event (e.g., praise and attention) or decreasing academic demands shortly after a problem behavior (e.g., hitting someone) might encourage the individual to use hitting again in hopes of getting the same results. In many cases these procedures can still be used if you wait long enough that the individual doesn't think you are doing them because he used problem behavior.
- Do not use these procedures in such a way that the person comes to expect that you will use the procedures every time that something upsetting happens. For example, you don't want him to start saying things like, "I'm mad. I didn't get to go swimming. Don't make me do work. That will make me feel better."

- Do not use the procedures if the individual has the skills to work through the negative setting events. For example, perhaps he has learned to successfully and consistently use a strategy to calm himself when he is disappointed (e.g., saying self-soothing statements such as, "I can handle this. I can wait until tomorrow."). If so, prompt him to use that skill rather than using these procedures. It is very important that the people with DS-ASD become increasingly independent. Teaching skills to help someone handle difficult situations helps him to become much more independent than just manipulating setting events for him.

- This speaks to a need for communication between the settings in which individuals are being served. For example, children with DS-ASD could have a back-and-forth book between home and the school. In that way, both settings will know of the times that they need to provide extra support.

For a fuller explanation of using setting events in this manner, see the article by Dadson and Horner in the Suggested Reading.

Keep 'Em Busy

One of the strongest tools for preventing problem behavior is keeping the individual actively engaged. Many people with DS-ASD are more likely to use problem behavior if they are not actively engaged in activities. This is not to say that we should keep an individual constantly engaged in activities. All people need downtime to relax; however, we should ensure that the individual has activities that he can do when he has downtime.

To keep an individual with DS-ASD actively engaged, provide him with more activities that require active participation than activities that only require passive participation. Examples of activities that require active participation include:

- walking in a swimming pool;
- playing a musical instrument;
- wiping down the tops of tables;
- vacuuming;
- walking;
- sorting silverware;
- dusting;
- making rags out of old clothing;
- shredding papers (e.g., bills) that need to be shredded;
- folding and putting away clothing;
- playing games with others; and
- engaging in conversation with others.

I prefer activities that require movement that requires some effort (e.g., moving arms and/or legs) and/or social interaction. The examples above do that. Some activities do not provide movement or social interaction to the degree that I prefer. For example, playing a game on an iPad or a computer requires little physical effort and seldom provides social interaction. Surfing the Internet also requires little effort and seldom provides opportunities for social interaction.

Examples of activities that require only passive participation include:

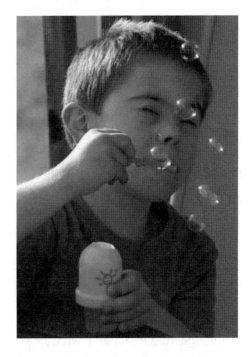

- riding in a vehicle;
- watching television; and
- listening to other people's conversations. (Please note that engaging in a conversation [i.e., listening and speaking] is active participation, while only listening is not.)

It is not that people with DS-ASD shouldn't engage in activities that only require passive participation, or that they shouldn't engage in activities that don't require much physical movement or social interaction. However, much more time should be spent doing activities that require active participation and include some physical movement and/or social interaction.

It would be best if the activities provided to the individual were functional activities and not "time fillers." Functional activities are activities that will help him to function more independently and to be productive. Examples of functional activities include: (a) setting a table; (b) putting away dishes from a dishwasher; and (c) folding and putting away clothes. Time fillers are activities that serve no other purpose than to keep the individual busy.

If the individual with DS-ASD has a short attention span, he will require relatively frequent breaks, or the activities will need to change often. In either case, work to slowly increase the amount of time that he is engaged in an activity before changing activities or providing him with a break.

Building Skills

Because much problem behavior is the result of skill deficits, often the strongest tool to help improve behavior is to teach the individual new skills. Because children and adults with DS-ASD often have many skill deficits, the skills to be taught should be prioritized. The skills that should be taught first are skills that are:

- immediately useful,
- frequently demanded, and
- decrease the individual's need to use problem behavior.

Perhaps the most common skill deficit that causes problem behavior is a deficit in communication skills. Imagine how frustrating it would be to want or need something but not be able to communicate that to others. Some individuals with DS-ASD have learned that, if they hurt themselves, hurt others, damage property, scream, or use other problem behaviors, someone will try to figure out what the problem is and try to fix it for them. After this happens a few times, the problem behavior becomes a strong tool for the individual to get his needs and wishes met, a tool so strong that the individual will not want to give it up.

In these sorts of situations, we should help the person learn to communicate his wants and needs in a more appropriate manner. This is often done through the use of **replacement behaviors.** Replacement behaviors are alternative behaviors/skills that will allow him to achieve what he is attempting to achieve through problem behavior.

I once was called in to provide recommendations for a man I will call Robert who was using severe problem behavior—specifically, he was smashing his face with his open palm so hard that he caused bad bloody noses that resulted in blood all over his face, on his hand and wrist, in his hair, and on his clothing. After some behavior detective work, I determined that, in essence, he was asking for food. Two people who worked with him said that sometimes they would give him a snack when he bloodied himself because it helped him to calm down. Robert's appetite usually woke up long after he did, so he often refused breakfast at home, but later, at about 10:00 or 10:30 at his day program, he became very hungry and began smashing his face. Apparently, at some point in his life, he had learned that if he smashed his face, he would get what he wanted, at least some of the time.

The intervention we used had three components. The first was to teach him a replacement behavior for asking for food; specifically, he was taught to use sign language. (He was unable to speak.) The second component was to provide him with some food prior to 10:00 so that he wouldn't need to use face smashing to ask for food. The third component was to never give him food when he smashed his face. This might sound cruel, but it was very necessary. If we gave him food when he smashed his face, it would encourage him to continue to smash his face in order to get food. It was also important because if face smashing never worked to get food and sign always worked, he would give up face smashing and replace it with sign much more quickly.

In the beginning of the intervention, Robert didn't smash his face much because we didn't let him get that hungry. When he did smash his face, we blocked his attempts. Later on, he quit smashing his face because he realized that using sign worked and smashing his face did not.

Teaching a Replacement Behavior

There are a number of principles that should be used when teaching a replacement behavior. Among them are the following:

- The replacement behavior should allow the individual to achieve the same results as the problem behavior did. If it doesn't, the individual will be unlikely to use the replacement behavior.

- In the beginning of the intervention, to the greatest degree possible, the replacement behavior should be effective every time the individual uses it. This will teach the individual the value of the replacement behavior more quickly, and it will result in a decreased likelihood that the individual will use the problem behavior.

  Please note that, over time, it will be important to teach the individual to wait until a more appropriate time for the replacement behavior to pay off. Some procedures for teaching this are in the section below titled "Teaching Patience."

- In the beginning, the replacement behavior should get the individual what he wants as quickly or more quickly than the problem behavior. If there is a delay in the payoff, he might not replace the problem behavior with the new behavior.

- To the degree possible, the problem behavior should not result in a pay off. If it does, the individual may continue to use the problem behavior. In the example above, face smashing no longer worked as a means to get food, so Robert quit using it. Using sign resulted in him getting food, and so he used it instead. When not allowing the behavior to be successful, you should be aware of a possible extinction burst, as mentioned earlier.

- If possible, the individual should already know how to perform the specific replacement behavior. For example if an individual has been using physical aggression to get attention, and the individual knows how to tap with a finger, he could be taught to tap the shoulder of a person from whom he wants attention.

  The value of using a behavior that the individual already knows how to perform is that the individual will have to learn only when to use the behavior, not both when to use the behavior and how to perform the behavior.

  Of course it is not always possible to find a replacement behavior that the individual already knows how to use. In those cases, if possible, it is best to use a behavior that the individual can learn easily. If the replacement behavior is too difficult to learn, the individual might not use it.

- If possible, the replacement behavior should be easier for the individual to perform than the problem behavior. In the example above, using sign to ask for food was much easier, and less painful for Robert, than smashing his face. The easier we make it for the individual to get what he wants, the more likely it will be that he will use the replacement behavior.

■ The specific replacement behavior should be one that a wide variety of people will easily understand and likely will respond to. For example, tapping another person on the shoulder to get attention is something that most people will understand.

It is important for us to teach skills that will allow children and adults with DS-ASD to integrate into society as much as possible. If only a few people understand the replacement behavior, the individual will have fewer opportunities to interact with others because hardly anyone will understand him. In addition, he might use the problem behavior with those who don't understand him.

The individual should practice the replacement behavior in situations that aren't difficult before using it in situations that are more difficult. This will allow him to learn the skill more quickly. For example, we did not wait until Robert smashed his face to start teaching him to use sign. We sat down with him when we thought he was somewhat hungry. We had small portions of food. Then, directly after one person prompted him to make the sign for food, another person gave him a little food. When he finished eating the small portion of food, Robert was prompted to use sign again and was immediately given another piece of food. Over time, he no longer required prompts. He had learned to use sign when he wanted food.

■ Until the individual no longer requires a prompt, he should be prompted to use the replacement behavior just prior to situations in which the behavior will be needed. It will be much more effective to prompt him to use the skill just prior to a situation than to remind him after the situation that he should have used the skill.

Teaching Patience

Patience is the ability to tolerate a delay for something without resorting to using problem behavior. For example, an individual doesn't have much patience if he asks for a glass of water, but then self-injures two seconds later because he hasn't gotten the water. Conversely, if the person asks for a glass of water and waits for ten minutes without using problem behavior, that person has much more patience.

Being patient is an important skill in society. Not everything can or should be supplied immediately when a person wants it. Being impatient can lead to more problem behavior. It will also limit an individual's ability to integrate more fully into society because that individual will not be able to function well in situations that require patience.

Teaching patience is very important if replacement behaviors are being taught. Generally speaking, replacement behaviors allow individuals to get access to something that is very important to them. For example, if an individual used self-injury to get food, getting food at that moment must be very important. If an individual learns a replacement behavior, it is possible that he will use the replacement behavior often and expect a quick payoff, too.

One way to teach someone to be patient is to ask him to complete a task before he gets the payoff from the replacement behavior. Initially, he should be capable of performing this task in a very short period of time—just a few seconds (e.g., you ask him to hand you something). After he successfully completes the task, praise him for completing the task and allow him to get the payoff for using the replacement behavior. As he becomes successful in completing very short tasks before payoff, gradually increase the duration of the tasks.

A second way to teach someone patience is to ask him to wait until you finish a task. Again, the length of the delay should be quite short initially, perhaps just a few seconds. Make sure that the length of the delay that he is expected to tolerate is very clear to him. For example, tell him that you will grant his request as soon as you are done putting away your book. As he becomes successful in tolerating a delay of a few seconds, gradually increase the duration of the delay.

A third way to teach an individual to tolerate a delay of reinforcement is to ask him to wait for a period of time before granting the request. When using this procedure, the length of time should be very specific and concrete. If the person can tell time, tell him what time his request will be granted. If he can't tell time or has difficulty telling time, use a timer that will make the amount of time concrete (e.g., a visual timer).

When using any of the above procedures, don't give the individual what he wants if he doesn't wait patiently. If he uses problem behavior, wait until he is no longer using problem behavior and has calmed down. Then prompt him to use the replacement behavior again. Decrease the length of the delay somewhat, but do not let him know that you are decreasing the length of the delay because of his problem behavior. This might only encourage him to continue to use problem behavior.

Consistency and Explicitness

Everyone who provides support to an individual with DS-ASD should be very explicit and consistent in all expectations they place on him. Being explicit will help him to know exactly what is expected of him. Being consistent with expectations will also help him to understand better what your expectations are.

Each person providing support to the individual should also be consistent in how they respond to the individual. In addition, all people providing support should be consistent with each other in how they respond to the individual. This will help the individual to understand better which behaviors pay off and which do not.

It will be impossible for everyone to be 100 percent consistent. However, please note that consistency will help the individual to feel more comfortable, and that inconsistency is likely to make him feel less comfortable and might result in an increase in problem behaviors.

When Meltdowns and Dangerous Behaviors Occur

It can be very frightening to be with someone who is screaming, breaking things, injuring himself, acting aggressively, or using other dangerous behaviors. In these situations, it is very important to appear calm. (It's even better if you actually are calm rather than just appearing to be calm; however, many people find that difficult if not impossible.) Responding to dangerous behavior in a frightened and unconfident manner typically results in the individual using even more difficult behavior. The person using dangerous behavior is probably upset, anxious, and not thinking clearly. If he realizes that you and/or others are frightened and uncertain, he may become significantly more anxious, making it even more difficult for him to behave appropriately.

The most important thing to do in these situations is to keep everyone, including the individual using the problem behavior, safe. The following are examples of some things that might be done to keep everyone safe:

- Move all unnecessary people out of the environment. That will help because there will be fewer people who can be hurt, and there will be fewer people whom the remaining people will have to protect.
- Having fewer people in the environment may also help the individual to become calm. Some people with DS-ASD have difficulty being around many other people even when they are calm. It can be much more difficult to be around other people when they are upset.

    I once worked with a gentleman for whom the most effective intervention during these situations was to leave him completely alone. Once he had calmed down, one or more support providers returned. The support providers never discovered any evidence of further damage to property or to him. Everything was as it was when everyone left.
- Take steps to help the person with DS-ASD to calm down:
    - Do not get close to the individual unless it is for safety purposes. Some people with DS-ASD who are upset can find it quite difficult to have someone in close proximity.
    - If you speak to the individual, speak slowly and in simple sentences. When upset, people with DS-ASD have even more difficulty understanding others. Speaking to them slowly and in simple sentences increases the likelihood that they will understand you.

- If you speak to the individual, speak reassuringly.
- Do not speak loudly or in a demanding/authoritarian manner. This can often lead to more anxiety, less clear thinking, and more problem behavior.
- If speaking to the individual seems to increase his difficulties, speak to him no more than is necessary.
- Minimizing the loudness of sounds in the environment can be helpful for many people with DS-ASD. Steps to take can include: (a) asking other people in the environment to be quieter; (b) asking other people in the environment to leave; (c) turning off things that are making noise; and (d) asking the individual to move to a quieter environment.
- Turning down the lighting in the environment can be helpful for some people. At times, light can be difficult for some individuals with DS-ASD. Do not make the environment completely dark, as that might increase the person's anxiety. Just dim the lights if possible.

If dangerous behavior occurs frequently, or if it occurs with great intensity, the people providing support to the individual should be trained in physical intervention techniques (e.g., restraint and escorts) by a qualified instructor. Physical intervention trainings provide instruction in how to physically manage an individual whose behavior is endangering himself or others. They can also teach: (a) preventative measures, such as how to calm an individual who is upset; (b) how to keep everyone safe without using a physical intervention (e.g., keeping a table between oneself and the upset individual); and (c) when to intervene physically.

Conclusion

It is important that parents and all others who provide support realize that people with DS-ASD are just trying to make sense of the world, and that they use problem behavior because it helps them to achieve important goals. Most individuals with DS-ASD don't have good perspective-taking skills, and therefore don't realize how their problem behavior affects others. Just like the rest of us, they are only trying to get their needs and wishes met.

Even though our lives are tough when children and adults with DS-ASD use problem behavior, it is important to remember that their lives are much tougher, not just when they use problem behavior, but all the time.

I have been in situations when someone is using problem behavior that makes me question whether I should continue to provide support to him. When I find myself thinking these sorts of thoughts, I remind myself why I am there. I am there to help the individual build skills so that he doesn't have to use problem behavior to achieve his goals. I am there to help him become happier. I am there to help him build the skills to enjoy the many pleasures of interacting with others and to help others enjoy the many pleasures of interacting with him. I am there to help him lead a richer and fuller life, a life that will be much better because of me.

So, when things get tough, remember why you are there.

Suggested Reading

Carr, E., Levin, L., McConnachie, G., Carlson, J.I., Kemp, D., & Smith, C. (1994). *Communication-Based Intervention for Problem Behavior: A User's Guide for Producing Positive Change.* Baltimore: Paul Brookes Publishing.

Dadson, S. & Horner, R. H. (1993). Manipulating setting events to decrease problem behaviors: A case study. *Teaching Exceptional Children 25(3):* 53-55.

Gray, C. *The New Social Stories Book.* (2010). Arlington, TX: Future Horizons.

Hodgdon, L. *Visual Strategies for Improving Communication: Practical Supports for Autism Spectrum Disorders.* (2010). Troy, MI: QuirkRoberts Publishing.

Wilde, L., Koegel, L., & Koegel, R. (1992). *Increasing Success in School through Priming.* Santa Barbara, CA: UCSB Koegel Autism Center. www.education.ucsb.edu/autism/behaviormanuals.html.

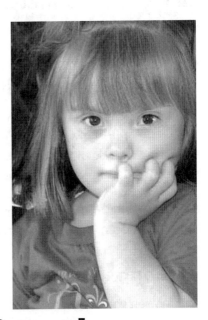

12

Designing Educational Programs for Students with DS-ASD

Patti McVay, M.S.

In this chapter, I want to share an overview of my many years in education in various roles, including assistant, teacher, special education director, and principal. I've been in hundreds of schools across the nation, and, while every school is unique, they all have the same goals and sense of opportunity and hope for the future.

Schools are centers for hope, community, and learning. Their role in our lives goes well beyond just buildings for learning. Along with parents, they shape the lives of the future and create vision for how we treat each other and contribute to our world.

When a school holds the belief in every child's potential, in their capabilities, and their value to the community, that belief permeates all that happens for kids. That belief creates belonging, high expectations, and learning environments that truly meet every child where they are and use the classroom and school community to provide instruction that increases every child's achievement. In schools where every child is valued, labels tend to fall by the wayside and the goal is for the classroom instruction to benefit every child rather than the child needing to fit the classroom.

School Communities

Every school has a wealth of possibilities to share with families, including those who have children with co-occurring Down syndrome and autism (DS-ASD). The key is getting a sense of the culture, values, and beliefs of the school in order to help plan for the upcoming journey. We'll talk more in the next few pages about how to discover those key school ingredients. After more than thirty years working in schools, I am convinced that relationships are key to making the journey as successful as possible for our children and I'll share more ideas about how to build those as we go.

Entering the School

When you walk into your school, what is your first sense? Do you feel welcome? Do people make eye contact with you? Do they say hi and offer to help or do they walk on by?

My friend Laura told me about all the spring days before her daughter, Sarah, moved from first grade to second. All but one of the second grade teachers would avoid eye contact when she walked by. They would pretend to be busy until after Laura was down the hall. At first, it hurt beyond words that their silent message was "I don't want Sarah in my class." But as Laura realized they were actually more fearful than mean, she took it as a challenge to engage them and share more about her daughter. Laura built many bridges that spring, and when Sarah moved into second grade, all the teachers began to see the child in Sarah, rather than all the labels. But the dilemma in all of this is that every day Laura learned she had to have her wardrobe of hats to meet all the people surrounding Sarah. Each day Laura packed all her hats and tools of each trade: mom, diplomat, teacher, advocate, advisor, activist, supporter, lobbyist, leader, architect, professor—knowing it was the way she would pave the path for Sarah's learning and success.

So, what if *you* get that "Oh no" feeling and teachers seem too busy or unwilling to talk or listen? Sometimes it takes persistence and other times it may take additional steps. You may need to:

- Bring a friend with you.
- Network with other parents about which teachers they have found collaborative and open.
- Enlist neighborhood friends to advocate for their children to be in classes with your child. They will do it because they see your child through their children's eyes.
- Check in with the principal (see the next section on School Leadership).
- Stay positive and persistent.

Usually you can find at least a couple of receptive staff. However, there may be times when you might run into too many closed doors and then it's time to pull together some friends and brainstorm the next steps. These may include things like:

- Checking out alternative schools that have a reputation for valuing all kids—again, following the same steps of reaching out to the principal first (see School Leadership).
- Checking with local Down syndrome and autism support groups for contacts within the school system.

School Leadership

The first instinct for most of us is to connect with the special education team at the school or with the district level special education administrator, but we now know from a great deal of research and experience that the first relationship to build is with the principal of the school. Principals set the tone for the school community and if they value students with disabilities, your child with DS-ASD will also be valued. I recently called a school to talk to the principal about a child who has a dual diagnosis. Initially, she was open and curious as to why I was calling. When she learned the child was receiving special education services, she immediately told me that I would need to talk to the vice principal, the special education teacher, or the district special education staff. Hmmmm . . . this is definitely a red flag.

If principals don't take ownership for *every* child in their school, then they aren't modeling that belief for the entire faculty. That's when our kids can get lost in the shuffle. So, it's time to dig deeper. If this happens with your child, this is a great opportunity to put on your diplomat hat and say, "I understand there are other folks I'll get to know when my son/daughter attends your school, but it's really important for me to get to know the leader of the school and to learn what your vision is for my child."

So, what do you do if you find out that the principal's vision is the opposite of yours, or, more often the case—the principal says all the right things, but you've heard that he or she doesn't follow through? First—if he has a view that is at odds with yours—it will be important to dig a little and find out what he does think of kids with disabilities. Often I find that there are "party lines" and sometimes it takes asking specific questions to really get a principal to open up about his view of our kids. Usually, a principal's hesitancies are founded in fear and in his own uncertainties, and this is when you realize you have so much to share with him. And that's why building a relationship with the principal is so important. Likewise, if the principal speaks about a similar vision, but might not be good at follow through, it's crucial for him to know you and your child and understand that you will be a positive force in the school for all kids.

Some folks will consider looking for a different school when faced with a principal with negative attitudes towards students with DS-ASD, but know that your neighborhood school will always be the ideal for the sense of community and belonging for you and all your children. But if there is no alternative, then it's best to get input from other parents and support agencies in the area such as Down syndrome and autism groups. Typically, the issue is that districts have special education programs in certain schools and our children are bused to those programs rather than bringing the appropriate supports to our kids.

Push on that door at your neighborhood school—use all your hats. Revisit the principal often, sharing both the good and difficult. Celebrate with him, encourage him, and—when appropriate—call attention to the good he is doing to the superintendent. This is just another way to teach people about the wonder of your child and pave the way for her success.

Parent Expertise

I can't say enough about the importance of valuing the expertise of parents. They know their children best and have thousands of hours and millions of minutes of experience. I mark their expertise in these measurements because their lives are not measured in the same way as I measure mine. Each day they awake, and their struggle, joy, difficulties, and adventure comes in the details of getting out of bed, getting through breakfast, and moving into the daily routines of going to school and all that awaits each day. Often, I've asked other professionals, my colleagues on IEP (Individual Education Program) teams, if they think they know more than parents, and some will definitely say "Yes." They say that their psychological, medical, or educational knowledge gives them that expertise, but then when I ask them, as parents, if anyone knows their own children better, they are quite certain that as parents they know their children best. Then they start to think a bit differently about other people's children.

Parents, please trust your instincts. No matter how much you know or don't know about DS-ASD, you do know your child. You know her likes and dislikes. You know her subtle and obvious forms of communication. You know what can make her smile, get angry, or become fearful or calm. You have a wealth of information to share with your school team. As you prepare to share your expertise with school staff, here are some ideas to consider:

- Share information and ideas through quick conversations and then follow up in writing.
- Write notes, cards, and letters about what you see that's good.
- Share weekend and family celebrations through photos that your child chooses and can share with friends and adults.
- Think of informal ways to share who your child is.
- In the formal meetings and IEPS, always follow up to be sure your insights, recommendations, and ideas are included.
- Some things to share with your child's teachers and other school staff who interact with her:
  - ❑ Your perspective of your child within the family—who she is as one of your kids, a part of the family—vs. defining her in terms of disability
  - ❑ Album of accomplishments, pictures, favorite places
  - ❑ Who your child is beyond school
  - ❑ What does and does not work for your child
  - ❑ Your child's strengths and successes

❑ Interests and favorite things
❑ Photos
❑ How your child contributes to your family
❑ Your dreams for your child
❑ Your vision for the future (just as with any of your children)

Building Relationships

Special education comes out of the medical model, which is very different than the educational model. When I understood that piece of information a bit better, it helped me understand how special education works within the school system. With the medical model comes the sense of the physician being the expert and driving the direction and all that happens, which means that special education began with that sense of folks in special education being the all-knowing ones about kids with disabilities. Traditionally, we kind of forgot the kid piece and focused in on the disability piece. But ideally we want to remember the whole child and bring together a team of people that keeps the whole child at the heart of the work. The education model began with a focus on educators as leaders and all knowledgeable and that we just needed to impart all the information to kids and the children needed to take it all in, no matter the mode of teaching or the individual learning styles of kids. But now we know so much more and know that when we create a learning environment that is focused on the many ways kids learn, we actually enrich the learning for all kids.

But what does this mean as we build relationships? As a special educator I was taught that I had the expertise in the school to work with kids with disabilities and no one else did. So, that empowered me to become the advocate and protector of kids and families—basically telling everyone else, "I know what to do with this child." However, what I have learned over my career is that a one-person "team" or a team with only special educators greatly limits the success of our children. Relationships that include general educators make a more robust team—with more heart and more ideas. Please keep in mind, however, that many general educators have been told that they don't have the expertise to work with children with DS-ASD and other disabilities. But the truth is, when teachers have a heart for kids, they are good instructors for all kids. And good teachers ask questions and keep learning. Inviting them to be a part of your child's team will enhance your child's success.

Here are some tips on building a relationship with general educators:
- Seek their input in relation to your child.
- Ask what strengths they see in your child.
- What would they like your child to learn?
- Help them value your child in their class. Ask them how they are including your child; how they value your child's contribution. Give them ideas on how your child contributes to your family.
- Ask what they think is important as kids develop friendships. How can they help make that happen for your child?

- Ask how you can support the teacher's needs—for time, training, and resources.
- Ask them what your child brings to their class.
- Do they know how important they are in your child's life? Tell them often the difference they are making, and, if there are difficulties, look for one good thing to focus on—to build on.
- Ask about their preferences for communication with you (mode, frequency, etc.) and establish a routine with them.

If the general education teacher refers you to others, remember this is probably because that is what their role has been in the past and why it's so important for them to know that you have faith in their expertise and really value their view of their child's learning.

As you build relationships with the rest of your team—special educator, speech pathologist, occupational therapist, physical therapist, school psychologist—keep in mind that if they give you the message (which I first gave my families) that I was THE one who had all the answers—it's a giant red flag. While it may be a comforting message because, in essence, it means that you don't need any of your hats, it's not true and it ultimately takes away the chance to build a wider circle of support. The best teams I've known included principals, general education teachers, the cafeteria worker, the bus driver, and the school counselor, along with the special educators.

Please don't misunderstand me—professionals who have chosen to work specifically with children with disabilities are often the cream of the crop. I know some of the best speech pathologists, physical and occupational therapists, and school psychologists in the country. They are my friends and make a difference in the lives of children every day, but the point is, the more diverse brains, hearts, and expertise at the table, the more benefit to your child and all children.

Team Roles and Responsibilities

In schools, we often make assumptions about who will do what. For example, the special education teacher always contacts the parents, the general education teacher always does the report card, the principal gets involved when there are difficulties, the paraprofessional does recess and bathrooms. It's really important to not make assumptions about who is doing what, and for you to know which team member to go to for key information and questions. Some of the questions to consider regarding team roles and responsibilities are:

- How is the IEP developed so all team members have input?
- How will I get information about my child's day from key members—such as the teachers, speech pathologist, or OT?
- Who is assuring that my child is accessing the curriculum successfully?

- Who is making the visuals that support my child's day? This can include schedules, Social Stories, contingency maps, problem-solving wheels, 5-point scales, if-then organizers.
- How does the whole team know how to use the strategies, visuals, and prompts that help my child be successful?
- Who is making sure data are being collected and that progress is being monitored and instruction revised when necessary? How often does that process take place?
- Who is training the team about Down syndrome and autism, collaboration, use of additional adults, inclusive best practices, etc.?
- Who supervises the additional adults and clarifies roles of paraprofessionals?
- Who works with all the students to create a welcoming, inclusive classroom community, sharing stories and role play about valuing diversity and differences?
- Think of other questions you want to know, then work with the team to write down the answers, so everyone has the same information and is in agreement.

Team Communication

Establishing a communication system with your team will help everyone be and stay on the same page. Some teams use a back-and-forth book with narratives only.

I suggest taking a few minutes with the team to brainstorm—listing what your family wants to know about the school day and then listing what school folks think would be helpful to know about home.

Then, if you are using a home-school book, put these key ingredients into an easy-to-use check-off system with just a few blanks for extra notes. Also consider using a "kid friendly" format so your child's friends can help fill it out. One teacher developed a system with a family that had pictures of all the weekly activities so that the student could circle the ones that took place each day (often with the help of a peer or adult). They also included who the child played with and his favorite activity of the day. Then the teacher realized she could use the system for all kids, and so at the end of the day, the class took five minutes to complete their half sheet of news. You can only imagine how well all the parents liked it!

If there are team notes or private things to be shared, the team may decide to use other ways to share those—through emails, weekly written updates, or phone calls. Some teams also use wikis and google docs—but it all depends on the purpose of the communication, and each team needs to determine what will meet both family and teacher needs.

Remember to use your common sense. If you want to know who your child is playing with or sitting next to in her classroom, it's best to go directly to the source—the classroom teacher. If you want to know how speech is going and what visuals are being used and how they can be generalized to classroom and home—again, go directly to the source and talk to the speech pathologist. The more direct the communication, the more you can help facilitate your child's education and success.

If your child is only in general education part time, it's still important to talk to the general education teacher and build that relationship because the skills that are learned in that setting and with typical peers are the ones that your child will carry into life beyond school.

In the Classroom

In this section, I'd like to share what both my experience and research say about creating successful learning opportunities for our students with Down syndrome and autism. Part of what we know is that the potential of kids with the dual diagnosis is

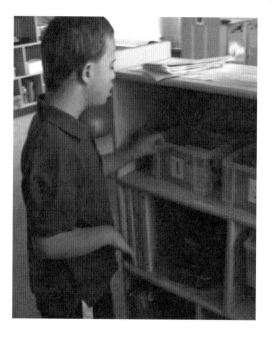

often hidden and lost because of what assessments don't measure and because the labels get in the way of people seeing possibility and setting expectations to match. Often I find that people immediately put kids with Down syndrome into categories of what they can and can't do without even knowing the child. It also happens to kids with autism, and so when we combine both characteristics, sometimes people aren't sure what to do.

As most of you know, it took years before kids with both DS and ASD were even "validated" with the dual diagnosis. One of my friends kept thinking she was an awful mom because all of the common knowledge about Down syndrome didn't fit her son and she was sure it was her fault. But she ultimately persevered, continuing to ask questions and push on the experts to finally discover that her son also had autism. She was both relieved and scared, but at least she now felt she had a path. In supporting her son and many other students with DS-ASD, here are some of the keys that I've observed:

- Visual supports—schedules, five-point scales, contingency maps, etc.—help. Visuals are so important because they provide ongoing and consistent information for students. They can include pictures, photos, and written words. They can be professionally done or a quick sticky note or cartoon drawing. They provide nonintrusive support and provide time to process information. Visuals enhance communication and organization and promote connections and interactions.

- Enlist typical peers in the development of visual supports—keeping them age appropriate and practical. Start small for a portion of the day, keep it fun, and use the interests of your child to promote more value and meaning.
- Find communication systems that work. Having multiple modes and ways for students to receive information and to express themselves is critical, but often we don't put enough systems in place: sign language, picture systems, verbal, and electronic devices (but only after an augmentative communication assessment has been done). It's best to try out a variety of systems first before investing the money in one. And it's critical to always have low tech backups when an electronic device is being used. This is also another place to enlist typical peers, helping them to learn how to use the systems and how to respond.
- Get augmentative communication and assistive technology assessments done to identify functional and relevant tools—do this early and continuously throughout school. Don't be afraid to ask for these assessments—in writing—to assure your child is getting the appropriate tools, support for the team to learn how to use them effectively, and consistent follow-up to be sure they remain the best tools as your child grows and learns.
- Ensure that the curriculum is modified and accommodated specific to this child—this is really important and not always as difficult as we make it. It's about starting with the curriculum that everyone else is using and finding the piece that makes sense to focus on for your child. It's about breaking the expectations down to smaller pieces. It's *not* about "dumbing" it down. Once a team learns how to make modifications and accommodations, they begin to see it benefits more than one child, because every classroom has diverse learners and there are no "typical" classrooms.
- Pay attention to positive behavior support planning. See the section coming up.
- Work with school staff to ensure your child has natural supports—reciprocal friendships and connections to typical peers, which includes working in small groups, partners, peer tutors, cooperative learning opportunities, class meetings, and role play, to name a few.
- Offer plenty of positive reinforcement—tangible, visual, and truly reinforcing rewards for behaviors you want to encourage—see more in the behavior planning section.
- Work with the school to arrange for team training—including parents—regarding best practices, knowledge of the individual's learning styles, teaming, defining adult roles and responsibilities, positive behavior planning, curriculum accommodations, modifications, and much more.

- Use Social Stories and perspective-taking tools—check out the work of Michelle Garcia Winner and Carol Gray.

- Try video modeling—taking videos of desired behaviors and actions to show your child the ways we act and do things. Consider reading *Seeing Is Believing: Video Self-modeling for People with Autism and Other Developmental Disabilities* by Tom Buggey and other sources that offer research-based best practices.

- Emphasize learning independent skills such as self-advocacy and self-monitoring, in order to prevent learned dependency and learned helplessness. The topic of learned dependency is of great importance, as I've watched very independent students become incapable of doing even the simplest thing because we taught them to depend on adults for cues and prompts. It can happen subtly and usually with the best of intentions because we want a child to know what to do—but in the long run, too much help can often lead to learned dependency. It's another reason visuals are so important along with the connection to typical peers. When a student is learning from many friends instead of one or two adults, her world expands and she learns how to be more independent.

- Data collection and progress monitoring will help assure that your child is growing and that the instruction provided is producing the results the team desires. The key to effective progress monitoring is regular review of the data to ensure adjustments are made to the instructional process when progress is faster or slower than expected.

- Encourage continuous whole team planning, problem solving, and celebration. When a team makes a commitment to ongoing problem solving, they understand that while we hope the plan we make will carry forward successfully for weeks and months, more typically, we'll need to make adjustments and rework things as we go and that is how life is. They don't blame problems or lack of progress on the child. It's never the child—it's about committed adults working together with a solution focus.

Inclusive Best Practices

Inclusive education is still an area of great struggle, but in my career as teacher, principal, and special education director, I've seen all kinds of placements and services for students with disabilities. I remain convinced that inclusion—done well with commitment, researched best practices, and heart—makes all the difference in the lives of our children.

Inclusion is about valuing every person, every child, and every student. Inclusive schools value every child by respecting and welcoming them, not just to be present in the general education class, but by setting up the necessary supports, services, and activities to build success. These include setting plans in place so that the child with Down syndrome and autism can be a successful participant and learner with a genuine sense of belonging.

So what about the times when kids need a space to go for pre-teaching, additional practice, remedial help, small group work, or individual instruction? That's when a Learning Center comes into play. Learning Centers are classrooms where any student can receive help or support regardless of whether she has a disability or not. So, rather than a separate place in the school for kids with IEPs, we now have a space that is viewed by all, kids and adults, as a place where everyone can get some extra assistance when needed.

In the Learning Centers I've known, kids come and go and the room is no longer tagged as the place all "those" kids go. Instead, kids may go there to take a makeup spelling test because they were out sick, or a high school mentor may help a middle school student with a science project. These kids may or may not have a disability—but the point is, all kids are getting their needs met while still having true membership in their homeroom class. They are no longer occasional visitors but have true belonging with their same-age typical peers—which is what we all long for.

Your school may not yet know about Learning Centers, so you may need to take the opportunity to share information about them and help the staff at your school research ways they can create similar learning environments for all students.

When I served as a postsecondary principal, the impact of inclusion for kids was made very clear. Students with varying disabilities including DS-ASD came to my program after their senior year in high school. I've always made a habit of meeting students before reading their files so that they could share who they were instead of my making an assumption of "knowing" them because I had read their assessments and reports. What I discovered was that I could tell who had been included in general education classes and who had not. The students who had been included were more social, more confident, more aware of the world around them and able to adapt to new environments. These students also had clearer interests and desires, which equated to more effective experiences and training to prepare them for life beyond school.

I am often asked about the terminology related to inclusion—which is why this section is entitled "Inclusive Best Practice," not "Full Inclusion" or "Partial Inclusion." Which then turns to the question—with all the evidence to support the benefits of inclusion, is it right for my child with DS-ASD? As described above, there may be times when any child needs a break or a time for pre-teaching or practicing a skill outside the general education setting in a Learning Center or the like. Ultimately, however, the goal is always for membership, belonging, instruction, and participation to happen with "MY" typical peers.

Recently I was asked about a child who was medically fragile and considered by most to be a child who didn't understand anything or respond to much and the question was wouldn't that child probably prefer to just be in a quiet room watching blinking lights and those kinds of things. I've been asked this a lot and have found that we often want to push away the things that scare us or we're not sure of. We know there is all kinds of research about the importance and critical nature of human contact, touch, and interaction for infants and the result for those in orphanages if they don't have it. So how could we possibly assume that it's better for kids to be isolated or separate? Do we need to be sure we have the right supports in place? Absolutely! Do we need to be sure our team is trained? Without a doubt! But the bottom line is making sure the plan is for what adults will do to support the child—not how the child should change to fit what adults want.

In the end, all the decisions that come your way will have to be weighed by what you know of your child and how all the decisions fit in your family and what you are able to do at any given time. The key is learning as much as you can, bringing friends along, maintaining high expectations, trusting that you'll get around the barriers, and doing what you can do today. Be gentle with yourself.

Building Friendships and Connections with Typical Peers

Recently I was talking to a long-time special education administrator about my experiences with high school kids with disabilities and typical kids developing

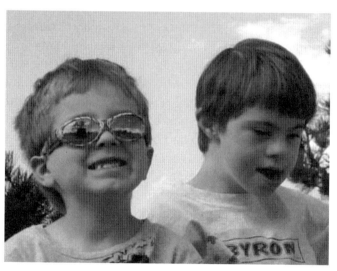

lasting friendships. I was amazed to hear her say that she didn't believe it could happen—she believed that kids with disabilities do better with their "own" type of people. Did that get your stomach just now—like it got mine at the time?

There are also some major myths about all kids with Down syndrome being happy, friendly kids and all kids with autism being loners, so where does that leave our kids with both? In my experience, all kids, all people, have that desire to belong, to be a part of a community, and to contribute from their very being. Here are some students I've known over the years:

Taylor: The first time I saw Taylor, he was in a special education class, hiding in a corner, self-stimming with a toy. His mom had filed for mediation, and, although he was only in preschool and not yet in our district, Taylor fell under my responsibility because he lived in our district. I observed during the morning, watching Taylor being pulled in and out of instructional lessons, chased and hit by classmates, and retreating whenever possible to a safe corner. The special education preschool had a reputation for being one of the best, with all the related and support services a child with Down syndrome and autism would need. Unfortunately, his mom didn't see it and neither did I.

We moved him to our kindergarten program to finish out the year. Quite suddenly, Taylor's whole world opened up and I never found him alone in a corner with only a toy. There were several kindergarten kids who were also learning how to play with each other and a few girls took a liking to Taylor, his blond hair, and bright smile. And through the remaining months of the year, Taylor and the girls became fast friends. Now, in second grade, Taylor is in a new school, in a new state, where inclusive practices are not even talked about because all kids are valued and what else would anyone imagine doing? He is building friendships, being valued for what he brings each day, really communicating for the first time in his life. His mom thinks she's found heaven.

Sarah: And how about Sarah and her second grade year? That was the year Megan and Sarah became really close friends. Megan's mom was dying of breast cancer, and, as the year progressed, I would often see Sarah and Megan off by themselves at recess, quietly talking and leaning on each other. One day when I was there visiting the class, I asked Megan about her friendship, and she said Sarah was her best friend because she kept all of her secrets. It didn't seem to matter that Sarah was basically nonverbal. Sarah did have a few words—one of them being "tail." And Megan was often called "Tail," meaning the best, because, of course, Sarah loved dogs and the tail was the best part of a dog.

OK, so most will admit, they can see friendships happening in elementary school, because kids aren't very sophisticated. But surely not in middle or high school. . . .

Shawn: In middle school, it was Shawn's student friends on the building committee who made sure that Shawn would be able to move through the school with his wheelchair. Sure, the adults would have come up with all the ADA requirements, but it was Shawn's friends who made sure his needs were personalized and counted beyond regulations. His friends saw him as a part of their class, their school—not a kid with a disability from that class down the hall.

Derrick: Derrick was a sophomore and the high school kids who joined his circle of support were as diverse as the school. Some were athletes or leaders, while others were into science and computers. Some felt as if this was their school, while others were struggling to have that sense of belonging. Initially the kids joined in for many different reasons, but in the end, it was having the opportunity to share space, activities, discussions, and getting to know each other that created the friendships.

Those friendships expanded beyond the school day because the high school kids had driver's licenses, enjoyed Derrick's company, and wanted to do what teenagers do. I remember the first time a group of friends took Derrick on the light rail system to a downtown farmer's market. Derrick's mom dropped him off and started to go through all the rules and supports and needs: "Remember to use the visual schedule and don't forget to read the Social Story on the train. . . ." Finally, the kids stopped her and reminded her that every day, Derrick shared their classes, sat through lectures, and worked together on projects, and that they knew him, cared about him, and just wanted to go and hang out. It was one of the longest days for Derrick's mom, letting him go, but also one of the best when she realized her son really did have friends.

If you've not seen "Voices of Friendship," please Google it and watch what some high school kids had to say about being friends.

Some things parents can do to promote friendship:
■ Make your home the place to be (welcome kids with snacks, games, and things your child and other kids enjoy).
■ Notice what other kids do—what they wear, where they "hang out," music they like, activities they enjoy.
■ Get your child involved in community groups and activities with neighborhood kids of the same age (scouts, camps, church groups).
■ Help your child reach out—phoning, inviting kids over or out to the mall or family outings. Invite two or three kids to keep things moving and help everyone build more friendships.
■ Show others how your child can participate and demonstrate ways to make your child feel comfortable and safe in new situations. Then step back and let the kids be together.
■ Keep adult presence and interference to a minimum in the day-to-day routine.
■ Speak up and get involved—let folks see you and your children in the neighborhood and community.

Some things teachers can do to promote friendship:
■ Have regular class meetings or circle time for sharing feelings and problem solving.
■ Use cooperative learning strategies with your whole class to teach communication and teamwork.
■ Set up buddy systems that facilitate students working with each other.
■ Go to students for solutions and ideas.
■ Role-play with all students to teach new skills and increase self-confidence.
■ Look for ways to involve every child in the curriculum—break down the task and let each child have a role using his or her strengths (using a calculator to check math work, being a timekeeper for a quiz, being a choir supporter by standing near a friend).
■ Make sure all students have the same opportunities with routines and procedures (homework, report cards, class presentations, awards).
■ Communicate and model your respect and valuing of the child labeled disabled through your interactions and behaviors.

Adapted from PEAK Parent Center, Inc.

Don't forget to include appropriate goals in the IEP related to cooperation and communication and friendship. For example, one of my favorite goals is for the student to learn to ask a friend for help before asking an adult, just as we expect every student in the class to do. We can't make friendships happen—but we can create welcoming classroom communities that foster respect and belonging and create a natural environment for friendship to grow.

Positive Behavior Planning

Over my career, I've seen lots of behavior planning and lots of processes to figure out the antecedents, frequency, and intensity of a child's behavior, and what I've seen in most outcomes are the same rote statements describing the reasons for a behavior as attention getting, avoidance, or gaining access to a particular object or activity. The missing piece that I've discovered is that we truly don't get down to what a child is trying to tell us. We make assumptions and miss the point. So what do we do? We need to take time to gather folks, including peers (if not in a meeting, at least giving them the chance to share their ideas through a class meeting or brainstorming) to come together and do it differently.

Finding the Real Reason behind Behavior: We often focus on the difficult behavior and what we will do when it occurs. But instead we want to focus on the specifics of the behavior. Instead of the typical statements of what it means, we need to put ourselves in the child's shoes and make "I" statements of what the behavior may be saying. There is great power in "I" statements. Instead of the process being adult driven, it becomes child centered. With clearer "I" statements, we can better plan what the need is and how to support the child.

An example: if a student is pushing things off the table or desk, our old way of thinking would be to describe the behavior as avoidance and noncompliance. But with "I" statements, we would consider some of these statements: "I don't understand what to do" or "I was told break was next" or "I want to play now" or "I hate math." With those statements in mind, the new skills and supports might look like: providing visual information before the activity, teaching the student to choose what to do after the task is finished, and teaching her to point to the picture of how I feel and what I want. It all becomes much more personalized and respectful.

You start to see that the outcomes are different when you try to look through the eyes of the child. You also start to see a theme—such as the need to know how to express feelings or to say what I want. Then it becomes the responsibility of the team to not only create the tools and visuals to give a student her voice, but also to be sure that tool is *always* available.

Listening to the Child: Recently I was observing a student with DS-ASD and everyone was telling me how excited they were that the student was using the communication system and that he seemed more engaged and communicative. And then, in the very next class, the visual system was moved out of reach while he was given work to do. He was upset and refusing. It broke my heart to watch the next few minutes as *no one* thought to give him back his voice, but only focused on making him do what was in front of him—though he clearly had something to say, as he was making sounds and pointing. Later, when I asked about it, I was told his communication system interrupts the class. And so I asked, "Do other kids talk in class? Do other kids use their voices?" The answer, of course, was YES. So why not this kiddo? Well, he always wants something other than the work we want him to do.

So we talked about how the effort to make this student do his work without his voice is disruptive, so why not start by giving him his voice? We talked about the rights of children to be able to use their voices and that it is tantamount to abuse to take a child's voice. The next question was whether the other students needed to learn when to talk and when not to and didn't this child deserve to learn that too. The other issue this situation called attention to was the perception that was provided to peers about how to treat this child with a disability and what to do if you don't like what someone is doing. This raised questions about whether their own voices could be silenced.

Collecting Data: Data collection is also critical—so that we know *when* things are happening, *who* is there, *what* the activity is, *what* the behavior looks like, and *how* everyone responds. It's important for parents to ask to see the data. There are very simple forms with those key headings listed that help paint the picture of what is happening. If the data don't give some clues, then we may not have enough data or accurate enough data. Parents can also collect data at home if they are seeing a concerning behavior. The more specific the data, the more information we will have to work through.

When behavior seems to be the biggest concern, the key is to ask for observations to be completed, for the team to track the questions listed, and then to get people together to look deeper. And parents—this is where you stand strong about your child being the very best kiddo ever and trust that the team needs to figure out what to do differently—what to add to supports or change—rather than ever considering that your child is the problem. An example of this is on the next page in Table 12-1.

The Role of Additional Adults—Paraprofessionals

I was a paraprofessional for seven years and had some great teacher models who inspired me to go on to teaching. The role of the para can be extremely difficult, with multiple supervisors and directions coming from every corner, along with a huge desire to do right by kids. So, as the team is planning for student supports, a crucial point to remember is that every team member has an important role and when the roles are clarified, the needs of students are kept in the forefront. When teachers understand the role of the para to be the classroom support, then the teacher takes ownership for every child.

Table 12-1: Sample of Collecting Data

What the child is doing— specifically detailed	Typical descriptors of what the behavior may mean	"I" Statements— personal descriptors of what the behavior may mean	New skills and supports
Pushing everything off the table	Avoidance, non-compliance	I don't understand I was told break was next I want to play now I hate math	Visual information before this activity Learn to make choices for what to do after I've finished this task Learn to point to the picture of how I feel & what I want
Hiding under the table	Over stimulated, non-compliant	I'm hungry I hid under the mat in OT today. It was fun	Learn to ask for what I need such as a snack or break Snack time within schedule Visual information about when OT is again and what the choices are now
Moving around the room during a lecture	Disruptive, non-compliant	I'm bored I need a break I don't understand	Modified curriculum Scheduled breaks Visuals & partner with a peer

Recently I was in a classroom and it was clear the teacher had ownership for every child. The para even introduced herself as a classroom para, so they understood how they worked together. As the observation continued, the para sat between two students with disabilities, helping them with lessons and moving to help others when they came to her. But then two students, at two different times, came to her and asked her which snack the student with DS-ASD wanted, rather than asking the student.

Do you see the red flag? The students without disabilities had come to believe that the para was there for that student and was that student's voice. It was not what this team wanted to happen, but it demonstrates the importance of looking for signs of what the para or extra adult's role is becoming. The other red flag that came up was that the students didn't need to do anything because the para was sitting with them. They didn't need to raise their hands, ask a peer for help, look for the teacher, or consider what to do for themselves, because if they looked puzzled or weren't working, this truly great para, with the best of intentions, would jump in and direct or prompt. It's the way learned dependency starts.

If, instead, a para moves around the class—helping all students, coaching peers to give directions or information—the scene becomes very different and we see student independence and confidence growing. That's why the role of the paraprofessionals and promoting student independence are so closely linked. We want paraprofessionals to see themselves as facilitators for students to learn to listen and focus on the teacher, to access the curriculum, and to check in with a peer. When paraprofessionals act as classroom paras, they refer parents to the teachers, follow teacher lesson plans, record progress data, help all students, and continually step back to promote student independence.

IEPs

Ideal IEPs are student centered, with a focus on the strengths of the student. IEPS serve as communication tools between parents and schools, giving everyone a chance to reach mutual agreement regarding the needs and goals of a student. They also serve as evaluation devices to monitor progress and are commitments of school resources. The main purpose of the IEP is to ensure that your child's needs are addressed.

Prior to the IEP meeting, it is important to ask about the agenda and timelines. Who will be at the meeting? What are the assessment results, progress updates, and proposed goals? Emphasize that you need to have time to read them prior to the meeting. You also may want to be sure that the agenda includes an opportunity for every team member to discuss your child's strengths, along with work samples and examples of the strategies and instruction that are helping your child learn. It's also great to ask for celebrations because too often the focus is on what kids can't do or what they are struggling with, rather than on their growth and success.

The model IEP should include: data about the student's present levels of performance and how progress is monitored. It looks at whether the goals change from year to year. If they are the same every year, the question is WHY? This IEP should include parent input, along with ideas, progress, and information from the general education teacher. Goals and objectives need to make sense, have meaning to the student, and be achievable. The goals should reflect what we want every child to learn. The goals should be tied to the core curriculum for the grade of the student and show how we will know when the goal is reached. They should also include goals that teach cooperative skills with kids without disabilities.

In IEP and Other Meetings

- Always bring a friend.
- Be respectfully assertive.
- Have your plan and be prepared.
- Take notes and ask questions.
- Ask for a break if things get tense or you just want to breathe.
- Take time to consider the information; it is OK to do so.
- Trust your judgment.
- Be a communicator.
- Acknowledge good efforts and intentions.
- Be a problem solver; you have solutions.
- Encourage brainstorming.
- Bring friends and supporters.
- Focus on solutions.
- Remind folks that it's about your child, not adult agendas.
- Offer ideas.
- Trust your judgment.

And When Things Are Breaking Down or Aren't Working So Well

- Go directly to the teacher and case manager.
- Write down specifics of what you want with timeline and give them a copy.
- Follow up with a thank you and copy key people—principal, director.
- If necessary, schedule a meeting with principal and director.
- Ask for an IEP meeting. Remember, by law, it is your right to ask for an IEP meeting at any time.

Transition Planning

When I think about planning for student transitions, I always refer to the "Open Letter to All" (2000) written by the People First of Oregon and Self Advocates as Leaders. They share their beliefs about what it means to be in control of their own lives, including being able to make decisions for themselves, being able to make mistakes, and living the life they want. They also believe it means being responsible and respected—just like everyone else.

They share that some of the things that get in the way of being in control of their lives are people who tell them what to do and make decisions for them, people who tell them "you can't" and people who don't listen to them.

They also share how professionals can help, and it starts with "inviting us to get involved and tell us what to expect." They request that others "ask us questions instead of telling us the answers."

These beliefs articulated by self-advocates are very important to consider as your child enters the transition years—roughly, ages 14 to 21. You will want to make sure that everyone involved in planning for your child's transition has a vision that is bigger than what life has been for most adults with DS-ASD in the past. Our young adults can go to college, live on their own or with roommates, have jobs of their liking, and so much more, and it's everyone's job to hold the same kind of dream for this child as they do for every other child. It means listening to the person, their friends and same-age peers, and giving them a way to voice their own hopes and dreams.

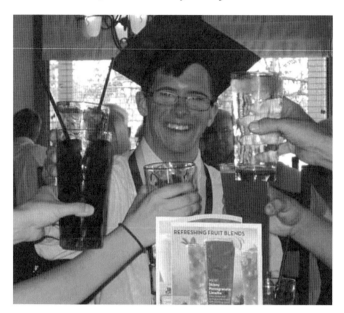

Part of the discussion about transition to adult life includes thinking about what happens in high school. There still remains a lot of debate about when to start thinking about jobs and vocational skills. When I'm not sure of which way to go, one of the key questions I ask myself is: "What are all the other high school students doing?" Are they doing off campus activities? Are they out of classes and away from their friends? And then I remember that high school only lasts for four or five years and that work goes on and on and on, so I recommend doing what we do for every other student and let them experience high school and learn all they can there because work and life beyond will always be there.

When looking at life beyond school for young people with DS-ASD, the view is really pretty bleak. While there are many systems in place, most are underfunded and offer few options. So it will be important to be creative and collaborative and gather as much information and support as possible. Person-centered planning is a really good way to plan, and it's critical to have a facilitator who is trained and experienced. Trained facilitators are hard to find, but keep asking—at the high school and at vocational rehabilitation and other local agencies. It's also important to know that just sitting around a table and asking the person centered planning questions and writing them on a paper to add to the IEP is not the same as having an actual planning meeting with all the key players— family, educators, community supports, business folks, and whomever you'd like to invite.

It's important to remember the plan is a work in progress, and, just as we talked about how difficult it is to be a team of one when kids are starting school, the same rule applies here—the more the merrier.

Celebration

Remember to play, rejoice, and enjoy who your child is and the uniqueness she brings. And don't ever let the labels, difficulties, and uncertainties take the joy of your child's presence from you.

Closing

More than anything, I hope this chapter has given you a window into schools and ways to navigate through them that might help make the journey a bit smoother. And so, here are some of the key items we've talked about that help create success as parents:

- Trust your instincts.
- Observe the culture and community of a school.
- See the principal as the key leader for your child's success.
- Create relationships with school staff.
- Develop team communication systems.
- Plan ahead and be prepared for IEP meetings.
- Understand the importance of your child's access to the core curriculum, accommodations, and modifications.
- Hold onto your dreams—keep high expectations for your child.
- Do your part to foster your child's friendships and connections to peers.
- Trust your instincts and your heart.
- Understand the importance of the modeling opportunities, friendships, and connections available with typical peers.
- Recognize the power of visual tools and how they will enhance your child's success throughout every day.
- Know how to use positive behavior planning processes that focus on what is being communicated through the behavior and the new skills to replace the behavior.
- Understand the role of additional adults, such as paraprofessionals.
- Remember that you know your child best.
- Use strategies and techniques that promote your child's independence while preventing learned dependency to learn the ways to carry the successes and tools from one grade to the next and from school to school.
- Plan for transition from school to life beyond.
- Celebrate often.

Please remember that you and your child are gifts to all of us around you.

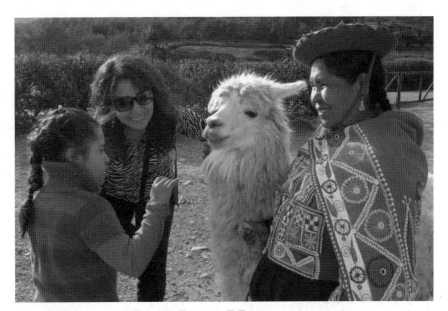

13

Multicultural Challenges
Co-Occurring Down Syndrome and Autism

Elina R. Manghi, PsyD, LMFT

Autism is a neurodevelopmental disorder characterized by impairment in three domains, including social interaction, communication, and restricted, repetitive patterns of behavior (DSM IV-TR, 2001). Recent epidemiological studies suggest that the incidence of autism is increasing. Such an increase may be due to the use of new assessment tools and better sampling procedures (Fombonne, 2003; Bertrand et al., 2001). According to the Centers for Disease Control and Prevention (2010), the prevalence of autism in the United States, meaning children having an autism spectrum disorder (ASD), has been estimated to be between approximately 1 in 80 and 1 in 240, with an average of 1 in 110. Autism has now become a national health crisis (Newschaffer and Curran, 2003), surpassing all other childhood disorders as the fastest growing epidemic in the United States.

Despite the enormous amount of literature available on autism, surprisingly little is known about the specific manifestation of the disorder and the appropriate tools with which to diagnose it within minority communities. Little is known about parental knowledge of appropriate interventions, the use of available resources, and/or the effectiveness of interventions among minority families. For those minority families who have children with Down syndrome and autism (DS-ASD), the difficulties are even greater than in the nonminority population, despite the fact that autism occurs in all races and nationalities.

As has been discussed throughout this book, the co-existence of Down syndrome and autism is of concern for many families due to the lack of professional knowledge regarding their co-occurrence. Through our work, we can say that DS-ASD also occurs in multicultural families. This chapter will review the difficulties faced by any minority family in the United States having a child with DS-ASD. A discussion of the obstacles these families must overcome will be followed by lessons learned through the activities of Grupo SALTO, the largest support group for Latino families who have children with ASD. Strategies by which to engage minority families in training and appropriate delivery models will follow.

The Problem

Although minority populations have grown significantly in the United States, they have not been represented in autism research, because up to now, most research data have generally been limited to Caucasian subjects. In one study of the racial differences in the age at which Medicaid-eligible children first received the diagnosis of autism, the researchers found significant racial differences with regard to the detection and diagnosis of children with an autism spectrum disorder (Mandel, Listerud, Levy, and Pinto-Martin, 2002). In a sample of children eligible for Medicaid in Philadelphia, white children first received their autism diagnosis at a much earlier age than African American and Latino children did. Additionally, African American and Hispanic children were less likely to receive treatment (Mandell, Boothroyd, and Stiles, 2003). More research is needed concerning the reasons for the general delay in the diagnosis of autism and the differences among the respective ethnic groups in terms of access to treatment services.

For many minority groups, mental illness and/or developmental disabilities are hidden. This is likely to occur due to cultural factors such as the shame and disgrace associated with admitting to emotional problems and the tendency to handle problems within the family rather than seek outside resources. Therefore, many minority families tend to delay the search for treatment until their problems become severe, which can lead to a lack of early intervention and the diminished efficacy of treatment.

Another issue pertains to the inaccessibility and incompatibility of the mainstream service delivery system, as typified by:

- inconvenient location of the facilities in the client's community with inadequate community outreach and organization efforts;
- a serious shortage of bilingual/bicultural service providers and a lack of efficient interpretation services; and
- the inability of mental health professionals to provide culturally sensitive, appropriate forms of treatment.

For example, many treatment and assessment methods for autism have not been translated from English into other languages. Consequently, communication difficulties and the lack of language-appropriate information concerning the nature of autism and the type of resources can discourage families from seeking formal services throughout the process of diagnosis and treatment.

The coordination of services and early intervention are critically important, since they are systematically planned and tailored to the needs and strengths of individual children and their families. State and local public agencies must coordinate efforts to ensure that minority children receive services without charge, or, at least, on a sliding scale. Due to scarce funding and a lack of knowledge as to the prevalence of autism among minority individuals residing in the United States, the available services vary drastically from school to school, district to district, and state to state. Many children in need of services end up on long waiting lists or possibly receive no services at all.

The demand for health services is strongly influenced by knowledge and information regarding those services. Thus, minority parents who lack information regarding autism, its diagnosis, and treatment may not seek services at an early stage. Moreover, professionals who serve the needs of minority families may not be adequately trained to recognize autism in individuals with Down syndrome.

Why Minority Families Are Underserved

Although training initiatives for autism have started to address the needs of families affected by the disorder, there has not been a consistent effort to include minority families. The deficit is partially attributable to the lack of trained professionals who are bilingual and bicultural or are able to culturally deliver such services.

Services for minority children with autism vary in terms of profile and quality, and usually they are provided in English. This leaves the parents isolated and unable to learn the appropriate interventions, which are essential for the development of children with DS-ASD. Minority parents report that few bilingual personnel are available in many of the targeted schools, which makes it extremely difficult for them to communicate with the teachers and special education teams.

It has been recognized that minority families generally have lower rates of mental health service utilization, prematurely terminate psychotherapy, and endorse unfavorable mental health-seeking attitudes (e.g., Atkinson, Lowe, and Matthew, 1995; Matsuoka, Breaux, and Ryukin, 1997). For example, one study found that the proportion of Asian Americans who used mental health services was approximately one-third of what might be expected, considering their population ratio (Yang and Wonpat-Borja, 2006). Families often delay using services until problems are very serious, so that more severe types of mental disorders are exhibited when treatment is finally used. Due to the severity of the problems when they enter treatment, the efficacy of treatment outcome may be diminished.

A cultural/financial barrier exists for minority families, given that many are immigrants with limited knowledge about the availability of resources. Moreover, the treatments that are available are too expensive for them to acquire without assistance. Therefore, given the absence of materials suited to the cultural needs of minority families, they will not be able to benefit from services and/or communicate with professionals who could otherwise help them. Other barriers identified in research include limited access to health services due to the lack of insurance coverage and/or a lack of knowledge regarding the co-occurrence of Down syndrome and ASD.

Grupo SALTO

In response to the needs of the Latino community in Chicago, Illinois, the author, together with a team of professionals in social work (Irma Hernández, LCSW), speech and language therapy (Pamela Bondy, M.S./CCC-L), and two parents (Matiana and José Ovalle), founded Grupo SALTO in 2004. Subsequently, it has grown to a membership of 400 Latino families who live in Chicago and surrounding communities. Grupo SALTO serves the needs of Latino families whose primary language is Spanish and who have a child or children with ASD. It is sponsored by the Hispanic Program of the Developmental Disabilities Family Clinic, Department of Disability and Human Development (DHD) at the University of Illinois, in Chicago. Grupo SALTO's mission is to provide state-of-the-art information, support, and services within a family framework that considers the culture of the family and community. Grupo SALTO is committed to bringing insight and hope to all aspects of life for the family that has a child with autism.

The main focus of Grupo SALTO is to provide training, education, and support to families of children with ASD. Monthly educational meetings include the dissemination of best-practice information regarding resources, interventions, and health issues for children with ASD. Additionally, we spend time with parents in order to help them learn the strategies that are necessary in order to take care of themselves and their other, typical children. Free childcare is provided through volunteers so that parents can attend the educational sessions.

Grupo SALTO also provides a program of creative expression for children with ASD, as well as their siblings. The program typically includes dance, art, and music. The goal of the program is to expose children with ASD to the arts while preparing them for inclusion in community activities. Sibling groups are available to help typical children address their concerns and questions in an environment that is safe and fun. A support group for teens with ASD is offered as well, thus providing opportunities to discuss life skills and the transition to adulthood.

Families that participate in the activities of Grupo SALTO not only report an increased knowledge of ASD but also enjoy the sense of community and empowerment that is part of their ongoing participation. Parents feel they are more able to speak out and educate community members about what it is like to have a child with autism. They also report a greater awareness and acceptance of other families who have children with disabilities. To that extent, they have been very supportive of Latino families with children with DS-ASD.

We, as a group, have earned the trust of our families by listening to their needs, by making the activities culturally meaningful, and by offering the services on Saturday mornings so that all family members are able to attend. Consequently, the growth of Grupo SALTO has been encouraged and facilitated. We provide snacks that are culturally acceptable, and we use visual systems, flyers, handouts, presentations, and other materials that are appropriate for our Spanish-speaking participants. We provide simultaneous translations when necessary, and we encourage parents to participate in different aspects of the organization based on their availability and willingness to contribute to the overall effort.

We have been very successful in having both parents participate in the various aspects of training. In turn, this has helped strengthen marriages while challenging the stereotypes of gender. We strongly believe in teaching our families the power of advocacy and leadership.

Intervention

It is well documented that children with autism, including those with DS-ASD, need intensive early intervention treatment. Moreover, autism treatment involves an interdisciplinary approach with comprehensive interventions, both at home and in school. Minority families who do not speak English do not receive adequate services due to the lack of trained, bilingual professionals who can share the cultural attributes of their communities.

The key to designing an effective mode of intervention for minority families is to first understand, respect, and appreciate their cultural diversity. Second, it is to make culturally relevant treatment approaches available to families with scant resources. Third, it is to use the families' strengths in helping them utilize the most effective strategies for handling autism within the home and within their children's own communities.

Accordingly, in response to the needs of the community, we created a plan to provide training to Latino families in Chicago who had children with ASD (including dual diagnoses such as Down syndrome and ASD). This training is sponsored by The Autism Program (TAP) and is delivered through the Department of Disability and Human Development at the University of Illinois, in Chicago. We developed two aspects to this training:

1. *Community Education and Training:* We provide direct training to community agencies and professionals serving the needs of Latino families. Training activities include an overview of autism, the co-occurrence of other disorders (e.g., DS-ASD), and common interventions for the treatment of autism. Each agency and participating professional receives educational materials translated into Spanish for dissemination among the Latino community. A consumer satisfaction survey is used to assess the effectiveness of training.

2. *Parent Education and Training:* We provide parent training to Latino families who have children with ASD, including dual genetic disorders. Training is conducted in Spanish. At the end of the parent trainings, we evaluate the training and encourage parents to discuss best ways to reach their respective communities. We assist parents who are unfamiliar with the assessment procedure so as to ensure that we obtain information regarding the training.

The parent training consists of ten weekly sessions offered at times that are convenient for families. Both parents and extended families are invited to attend the training sessions. The first three sessions are group-oriented, followed by six individual sessions, and then the last session, which is again given in the group context. In each cycle we train six families. We prefer to train families immediately after they receive the diagnosis of ASD; however, we also teach families who have never received this type of training despite having received the diagnosis of ASD in the past.

The group sessions are designed to teach the most effective interventions to deal with the learning, behavioral, and sensory problems associated with ASD. Families get to know each other, and consequently they embark together on a path that will lead them to a better understanding and acceptance of their children's conditions. Cultural beliefs and barriers are discussed, as they are important elements in the success of any training. During the last group session, we assess progress and we train parents to work with their children's school. Finally, we talk about the importance of taking care of oneself and explore the essential strategies for stress management.

The individual sessions are tailored to the specific needs of each family. During these sessions the parents are able to practice what they have learned during the group sessions. We use visual systems that are culturally appropriate. We teach parents how to implement behavioral interventions that are successful, and, of course, appropriate to the families' cultural beliefs. We help parents identify what prevents them from successfully applying appropriate interventions, and together with them we celebrate every success, no matter how small it might be.

Parents are encouraged to participate in the training sessions offered by Grupo SALTO as described above. The sessions provide parents with another avenue by which to connect to a community of peers and at the same time continue their learning. We view parents as mentors who will not only help their own children, but can also help other families that are just starting.

The role of the trainer is to help families attain a new perspective, and, at the same time, to promote creativity within the group. The trainer must therefore help the participants avoid failure. This is important because children who have ASD are constantly confronted by the experience of failure. When parents learn to recognize the signs and plan strategies that will help their children avoid repeated failure experiences, behaviors and family life will both improve. By learning to recognize what leads to their own experience of failure, parents will be more fully prepared to do the same with their children. Additionally, the trainer facilitates connections among parents, helping them break the cycle of isolation.

What We Have Learned

It is very important to avoid the bias of presupposition. This is particularly true, given the knowledge that minority families are able to benefit from training and can be very successful in applying interventions that work for their children. However, they usually come to training with a lack of current knowledge regarding the management of ASD. They may believe there is little that can be done to improve their children's functioning (which might have been the case in their country of origin). Furthermore, due to language barriers they may have been unable to access current information. Many of our families may not have easy access to the Internet or, because of language barriers, they may not be able to discern the appropriate intervention based on best practices.

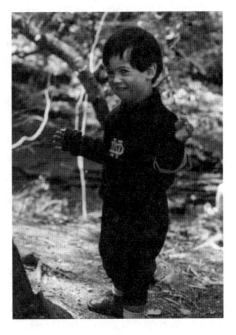

We strongly believe the success of our training lies in the way we present our material, which is easily understood, visually accessible, provided in the family's first language, and accompanied by videos that demonstrate the concepts. The ability to conduct hands-on training also plays a role in the success of implementation. We ask both parents to work on creating visual schedules or a library of photos to use at home and in the community. We help them create behavioral plans with which to address particular problems they are experiencing as families. We work closely with each family member to help all of them be successful in implementing the program. We create an emotional space where families are able to discuss their fears and concerns.

Factors that influence the success of training include the level of family stress, the family's attitude toward change, the strength of the parental relationship, and the trainer's ability to understand what cultural factors might obstruct the ability to apply the interventions presented. Occasionally, we have encountered families that were very resistant to the use of behavioral interventions. For example, many minority families view the use of rewards as bribery and a method that is not congruent with their belief systems. Unless the trainer is able to address this issue from a cultural perspective and show families the distinction between a reward and what would be considered bribery, the intervention will not be effective.

If the family is experiencing high levels of stress, which might not be related to their child's disability, it may be very difficult to learn and implement new techniques. Therefore, initially we advise the family in order to reduce stress, and then we focus on the intensive learning.

We carefully tailor our program to meet the needs of the community. Sessions are scheduled at times that are most convenient to families, in a central location that is readily accessible by public transportation. For some of the training sessions we are able to provide childcare.

Initially, we had questions regarding the success of a training that included Latino parents whose children had either ASD or DS-ASD. However, we discovered that there were benefits to this arrangement. First, parents were able to understand that ASD can occur along with other conditions. Second, because the training focuses on the behavioral management of difficulties associated with ASD, the content of each session is clearly applicable to both groups. Third, parents have been able to express support for the parent of a child whose condition is more complex. Finally, an important discussion took place in which we addressed the difficulties of: a) someone who has readily been identified as having a disability due to obvious physical features, as is the case of children with Down syndrome; and b) someone who has not been easily seen as an individual with a disability, due to the lack of obvious physical features.

We recently developed a program for Polish families who have children with ASD. The first family we trained has a nine-year-old child who had been diagnosed with DS-ASD. He had very poor communication skills and a series of sensory issues, and was not toilet-trained. We used a "train the trainer" model in which the author trained a Polish mental health provider to implement the ten-session program. The author presented the material in English, and the Polish mental-health provider translated the content to the parent. We used visual systems to address the toileting and communication difficulties. The mother was very enthusiastic about trying the program, and she proved very successful in toilet-training her child. With support, the teaching of basic behavioral principles, and use of visual systems, her child is beginning to communicate his needs. Temper tantrums have diminished significantly. Currently, we are completing the translation of the manual into Polish so that we can continue to assist the community.

The Asian American community is another underserved group in Chicago and elsewhere. We are developing a project to provide educational training regarding autism to Asian American frontline professionals in Illinois as well as parents/families in appropriate languages (Chinese, Korean, and Lao). Additionally, through these training sessions we will examine the unique needs of Asian Americans' parents/families that might be affected by autism. Training and evaluation will bring awareness to the importance of detection, diagnosis, and treatment for children with autism spectrum disorders, including DS-ASD within Asian American communities.

The approach we take in developing culturally appropriate interventions is always to be informed by the community about their needs, the best way to approach families, their understanding of services, their definitions of mental-health issues, and how one can get well within his or her own culture.

The following is a guide to working with three multicultural family groups. This guide is meant to be informative about some of the most salient values and beliefs of these ethnic groups, but should in no way be considered exhaustive. There are many individual and family differences within each group, as determined by socioeconomic status, education, place of origin, etc. These guidelines have been adapted from the *Cultural Competence in Autism Training Manual* (Manghi, E., Montiel, F., and Philips, D., 2010).

Considerations in Working with African American Families

Values, Beliefs, and Life Ways

- Strong kinship bonds;
- Strong religious orientation;
- Large percentages of African American families are headed by single parents;
- Adaptable family roles;
- Use informal support network; e.g., church or community;
- Distrust of government and social services;
- Most are assimilated into the Anglo-American culture;
- May not like to admit they need help, given a strong sense of pride;
- May lack knowledge about available services and how the system works;
- Natural remedies used frequently; e.g., prayers for the sake of healing;
- Seniors are highly respected, as aging represents respect, authority, and wisdom;
- May tend to keep things hidden within the family system; difficulty reaching out;
- Poverty impacts education, self-esteem, quality of life, and lifestyle throughout one's lifetime.

Intervention Tips

- Familiar with Anglo-American communication patterns;
- Show respect at all times: a history of racism and sense of powerlessness
- Impacts interactions;
- Prolonged eye contact may be perceived as staring and interpreted as confrontational or aggressive;
- Use community and/or religious leaders if assistance is needed;
- Do not use "street slang," which could be interpreted as disrespectful or offensive;
- Do not address by first name unless requested to do so, since it could be considered disrespectful;
- May not like to be asked questions about finances, past relationships, or marital status; initially it is more important to gain trust.

Considerations in Working with Latino Families
Values, Beliefs, and Life Ways
- The group has more importance than the self (collectivistic);
- Strong family unity; respect for and loyalty to the family;
- Strong spiritual and religious orientation;
- Distrust/fear of "government"; immigration status may impact interactions;
- Male (machismo)-dominant; father/husband may be the primary authority figure;
- Age-dominant; respect for hierarchy;
- Live for the present/today, fatalistic; a perceived inability to control the future;
- Take care of their own;
- Negative view on asking for help; can take time before an agency is trusted;
- Modesty is important;
- Majority is Catholic; church is seen as a source for services and information;
- Strong belief in the importance of prayer;
- Very proud of heritage; never forget where they came from;
- Comfortable with physical contact (hand shaking and hugging).

Intervention Tips
- Respect is basic for all communication;
- Like to be approached first; do not easily initiate conversation;
- Eye contact is perceived as a more confrontational body language than a sign of respect;
- Being ignored is a sign of disrespect and can be perceived as offensive;
- Being personal, warm, trustworthy, and respectful is valued;
- Avoid too much gesturing;
- Encourage the individual to ask questions;
- Make sure your questions have been understood, given the general reluctance to ask questions;
- Maintain an accepting attitude;
- Let them know their ideas, thoughts, etc., are valued;
- Less personal space is needed than with Anglo-Americans;
- Very expressive in their communication; seek physical contact; e.g., handshaking and hugging;
- Determine level of fluency in English; use an interpreter if necessary;
- Do not like to be asked about immigration status, religion, or financial sources.

Considerations in Working with Asian Families

Values, Beliefs, and Life Ways

- Need to maintain harmony within the group;
- The group has more importance than the self (collectivistic);
- Respect for hierarchy;
- Age-dominant;
- Male-dominant;
- Pressure to "keep face";
- Overt displays of emotion are considered shameful;
- May tend to keep things hidden within the family system; difficulty seeking services.

Intervention Tips

- Gather information regarding specific families' ethnic backgrounds, languages, immigration and refugee experiences, acculturation levels, and community support systems;
- Develop trust by establishing and adhering to rules of social conduct and proper social interaction;
- Attempt to maintain, and, if appropriate, reestablish traditional family structures according to cultural norms;
- Respect the family hierarchy;
- Use extended family members for support systems; lines between nuclear families and extended families are not as rigid in Asian families as they are in Western culture;
- Allow families and their individual members opportunities to "save face" whenever possible;
- Avoid creating situations that may lead to conflict and confrontation, and instead use indirect methods of communication, when appropriate, to make a point;
- Because Asians prefer to keep problems within the family, confidentiality is critical; families must be assured that their problems will not become public knowledge;
- Service providers must be active and offer tangible interventions for Asian American clients, as passivity in the worker may be viewed as a lack of expertise and authority; many Asian American families seek concrete, tangible solutions to their problems and are uncomfortable with process- and insight-oriented strategies.

For All Families Regardless of Ethnic Background

- Consider educational level—written and spoken words should be adapted to level of understanding;

- No cultural group is homogeneous; one must consider within-group differences;
- Individual and subgroup differences exist in every culture;
- Family, as defined by each culture, is usually the primary system of support and is the preferred intervention;
- Families/clients are the ultimate decision makers for services and support for their children and themselves.

Intervention Tips for Minority Families Who Have a Child with DS-ASD

- Develop interventions, such as visual systems, that are culturally appropriate;
- Gain an understanding of the family's definition of autism, and if necessary, offer a different way of viewing the disorder;
- Educate families about autism, its diagnosis, and treatment;
- Expand the family's support;
- Engage community support (e.g., church, school, park district, etc.);
- Encourage independence within the family's cultural comfort;
- Future planning: if appropriate, engage extended family and community support, and encourage communication between the family and other service providers;
- The provider may act as the bridge between cultural beliefs.

None of the above interventions would be possible without a culturally competent organization to provide the corresponding services. Therefore, the organization that is culturally competent will have a defined set of values and principles, as demonstrated by behaviors, attitudes, policies, and structures that allow it to work effectively cross-culturally. Consequently, systems of care that are able to provide multicultural services value diversity (instead of simply tolerating it) and thereby adapt to the cultural context of the communities they serve. Cultural competence is a developmental process that evolves over time. What is important is that organizations incorporate diversity into all aspects of policy-making, administration, practice and service delivery, systematically involving consumers, stakeholders, and communities (Cross et al., 1989).

Conclusion

In summary, in order to plan for culturally diverse families affected by DS-ASD, it is imperative that we look into culturally appropriate treatment models. Minority families are as eager to help their children with disabilities as mainstream families are. Inadequate schools, unresponsive medical systems, socioeconomic obstacles, lack of adequate training, and language-related issues combine to disturb the stability and sense of control that minority families could otherwise have (Montalvo and Gutier-rez, 1990). The challenge is to develop and implement strategies that can address the specific needs of minority families who have children with DS-ASD and who are a minority group within the Down syndrome population, and, in turn, within the general society. By facilitating services, understanding the cultural needs of each family, and providing the interventions that we know work, we will have children and adults with DS-ASD who are better adjusted and more productive members of society.

References

American Psychiatric Association. (2000). *Diagnostic and Statistical Manual of Mental Disorders.* 4th ed., text rev. Washington, DC: American Psychiatric Association.

Atkinson, D. R., Lowe, S., & Matthews, L. (1995). Asian-American acculturation, gender, and willingness to seek counseling. *Journal of Multicultural Counseling and Development 23:* 130-38.

Bertrand, J., Mars, A., Boyle, C., Bove, F., Yeargin-Allsopp, M., & Decoufle, P. (2001). Prevalence of autism in a United States population: The Brick Township, New Jersey, investigation. *Pediatrics 108(5):* 1155-61.

Cross, T., Bazron, B., Dennis, K., & Isaacs, M. (1989). *Towards a Culturally Competent System of Care, Volume I.* Washington, DC: Georgetown University Child Development Center, CASSP Technical Assistance Center.

Fombonne, E. (2003). The prevalence of Autism. *Journal of the American Medical Association 289(1):* 87-89.

Mandell, D. S., Boothroyd, R. A., & Stiles, P. G. (2003). Children's use of mental health services in different Medicaid insurance plans. *Journal of Behavioral Health Services & Research 30(2):* 228-237.

Mandell, D., Listerud, J., Levy, S., & Pinto-Martin, J. (2002). Race differences in the age at diagnosis among Medicaid-eligible children with autism. *Journal of the American Academy of Child and Adolescent Psychiatry 41(12):* 1447.

Manghi, E., Montiel, F., & Philips, D. (2010). *Cultural Competence in Autism Training Manual.* Training program developed for the Autism Program of Illinois (TAP).

Matsuoka, J. K., Breaux, C., & Ryujin, D. H. (1997). National utilization of mental health services by Asian Americans/Pacific Islanders. *Journal of Community Psychology 25:* 141-45.

Montalvo, B. & Gutierrez, M. J. (1990). Nine assumptions for work with ethnic minority families. In G. W. Saba , B. M. Karrer, & K. V. Hardy (Eds.), *Minorities and Family Therapy.* New York, NY: Haworth Press.

Newschaffer, C.J. & Curran, L.K. (2003). Autism: An emerging public health problem. *Public Health Reports 118(5):* 393-99.

Yang, L.H. & Wonpat-Borja, A. (2006). Psychopathology among Asian-Americans. In: F.T.L. Leong, A.G. Inman, A. Elbreo, L.H. Yang, L. Kinoshita, & M. Fu (Eds.), *Handbook of Asian American Psychology.* Thousand Oaks, CA: Sage.

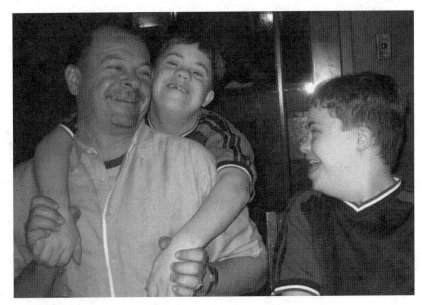

14

Life Planning for Individuals with DS-ASD

Hal Wright, CFP®, LPL

As a parent of an adult daughter with Down syndrome, and as a Certified Financial Planner, I can tell you that special needs planning is not easy; in fact, it can be quite challenging. It can feel a bit like trying to put together a jigsaw puzzle. The best way to start putting together a puzzle is to look at the picture on the box. Then, you find the major pieces—the corner pieces and the pieces that make up prominent features in the center. What I hope to achieve in this chapter is to show you the picture on the box of "Life Planning," and help you identify the key pieces so you can start planning for your child's future.

Special Needs Planning

The purpose of special needs planning is to create the best quality of life for a person with a disability, appropriate to his or her needs and capabilities, what they want for themselves, and what the family can afford. A comprehensive special needs plan integrates four elements of special needs planning:

> *1. Life Plan*—Life planning envisions a quality of life for your child, the child's rightful place in the community as an adult.

2. *Resource Plan*—Resources make the life plan possible. Resources will come in two flavors—government supports and services to the extent the individual is eligible, and "private pay" to the extent the family can afford.

3. *Financial Plan*—Financial planning is about how to pay for the resources while preserving eligibility for government assistance. You will need an estimate of lifetime financial support and how that support can be provided. Usually, a special needs financial plan will include a plan to establish, fund, and manage a special needs trust.

4. *Legal/Estate Plan*—Legal or estate planning involves executing the legal documents to assure that your child is protected and that your wishes are carried out when you die. The legal documents typically include wills, appointments of persons to hold powers-of-attorney and health-care directives for both parents; and, in most cases, a special needs trust.

Life Planning

A life plan typically addresses the following:
- The circles of family and friends bound by love and not pay
- Professionals to fill the roles not taken by family and friends
- Social and recreational activities
- Spiritual needs; participation in a religious community
- Independence to the extent of one's capabilities
- Perhaps a job or business one can be proud of
- A suitable residential environment
- Special needs—physical, psychological, medical, and safety

A key component of life planning is an annual Individual Life Plan (an ILP). An ILP is simple in concept, though not so easy in practice. Basically the steps are:
- Form a team
- Get a facilitator
- Assure participation and input from the person with special needs
- Decide on questions or goals the team is to address
- Hold the meeting; develop goals and an action plan for the year
- Status progress
- Repeat the following year

Guardianship

One decision parents will face is whether to petition a state court for guardianship when the child turns 18. Guardianship is not a social relationship between parents and a child. It is a legal concept under which the State asserts its power to protect minors, those too young to take care of themselves, or those incompetent to do so because of a disability. The State assumes that parents are the appropriate guardians for their minor child. Once children reach the "age of emancipation," they are old enough, theoretically, to take care of themselves. In almost all states a child becomes an adult on his or her 18th birthday. The parents' roles as guardians then cease unless a court of law finds it is in the child's interest to have those roles extended. Parents, if they wish to continue as guardians after the child turns 18, will need to petition a state court for appointment. A person for whom a guardian has been appointed is legally known as a "ward" of the guardian.

In most states you don't need an attorney to file a guardianship petition. You can do it yourself if you file the proper forms and pay the fees. However, consult with an attorney if the appointment is likely to be contested.

In most states you can petition for full or limited guardianship. Under full guardianship, the guardian has the authority to make decisions for almost all aspects of the person's life. Limited guardians are given authority over specific aspects (defined by the court) typically for financial and legal affairs.

The purpose of guardianship is to protect the individual and to allow someone to make decisions that an individual cannot make safely or competently for himself or herself. It also allows the guardian a "place at the table" with medical, government, and professional people when decisions are made for the individual. Guardianship gives the power to initiate or intervene in legal actions and perhaps to appeal a denial of government benefits or civil rights actions. It also allows someone to take steps to prevent the ward from being exploited by others.

An appointment of a guardian takes away the rights of an individual to manage his or her own life or defined aspects of it. These rights can include the right to make decisions such as where to live, to make major purchases, to travel, to incur debt (e.g., have a credit card), etc. It can also include the right to make medical decisions, and— in some states—the right to vote. Because guardianship is a taking of someone's right to manage their affairs, it should be done only when necessary, when lesser forms of protection are inadequate.

There are alternatives to guardianship. These include naming someone to be an advocate or advisor, appointing someone with power-of-attorney, designating someone as a representative payee for Social Security benefits, and authorizing someone to have access to records otherwise shielded by privacy protections, e.g., medical files.

Should you petition for some form of guardianship for your child with DS-ASD? Carefully consider his or her ability to make decisions and need for protection. Seek the least restrictive form of protection. However, parents typically err on the side of protection. Guardianship can always be amended or revoked by a court. If you are appointed as full guardian and experience proves that to be unnecessarily restrictive, you should petition the court to have the guardianship narrowed to only the necessary needs or terminated.

Transitions

Life planning should focus on the major transitions from one phase to the next to assure that your child will come through them safely and wind up in a stable situation. Although theoretically you should always be planning for the child's lifetime, practically you will give most attention to the next major transition. I advocate life planning at the following stages:

- **For the newborn or minor child**—Have adequate insurance for the death or disability of one or both parents. Execute wills to name successor guardians should you both die together. Have a family financial plan.

- **When the child is in late middle school**—Focus on the child's situation after aging out of school, life skills coaching, perhaps preparation for employment. At this stage you should develop a comprehensive special needs plan including life, resource, financial, and legal plans.

- **In the transition years before the child ages out of school** (the late teens)—Focus on employment potential, continuation of services for special needs, and the long-term residential situation. Update your special needs plan and assure you addressed affordability.

- **In the child's twenties,** if he or she is to transition out of the parents' home, either into a state-provided or private residence—Update the comprehensive special needs plan; develop a detailed estimate of lifetime support; verify that there is sufficient family wealth and/or life insurance to pay for the resources that enable the life plan. If the plan is not affordable, the life plan must be scaled back.

At all stages of your child's life, you should have a contingency plan in case one or both parents die or become unable to provide or care for their child. Assure that those in the circles of lifetime support have been identified—family and professional—or how these circles will be filled when needed. If hiring professionals is part of your plan for supporting your child, verify there is sufficient family wealth or insurance to pay for their services.

Review and update the plan when there are significant changes in your life or your child's. You should plan for each transition and update your plan after the transition. But there are other changes you may need to address. These changes can involve a change in circumstances such as a change in medical condition, the family relocating to another state, or changes involving available resources. It can be changes in a child's finances, such as a monthly Social Security Disability Income (SSDI) replacing the Supplemental Security Income (SSI). It can be changes in a child's legal situation—the parents' divorce, for example. You should watch for circumstances when items of income or expense start or stop or change significantly.

There are also changes in the lives of parents or family that can require reassessment of the special needs plan. The changes may be the birth of a new sibling or a sibling entering or leaving college or leaving the family nest. It could be a parent's change in employment including promotion, job loss, relocation, or retirement. It could be a parent's disability or major illness. Even if the family situation is stable, a special needs plan should be reviewed at least annually and updated if needed.

Resource Plan—Government Assistance

Federal Government Programs

Families need to understand that it is government policy to provide for only the most basic needs of an individual with a disability—life maintenance, essential health care, and support at the poverty line (in many states, not even that). Basic assistance is

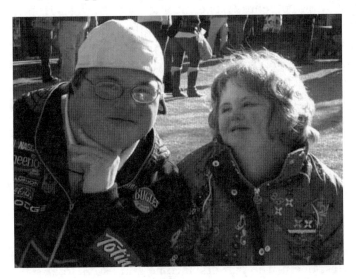

for food, shelter, health care, job assistance, and someone to manage government services. It's what's known derisively in the advocacy community as "eats and sheets." Don't believe it? Look at the numbers. The national poverty guideline published by the U.S. Department of Health and Human Services for 2012 is $11,220 per year, $935 per month. For 2012, Supplemental Security Income, the sole source of financial assistance for many people with disabilities, is $698 per month, 75 percent of poverty level. What gets a person with a disability to the poverty line? It may be food stamps, low income housing assistance, and low income energy assistance. It gets no better than that.

At the federal government level, there are two forms of assistance—cash payments and health care. With each, there are two types of programs— "entitlement" and "need-based." Entitlement programs are insurance programs. One is entitled to benefits because one (or one's parents or spouse) paid the insurance premiums, i.e., taxes. Need-based programs are programs intended to help a person who cannot pay for his or her basic needs. To qualify for a need-based program, one's income or financial assets cannot exceed very low dollar limits. One must be poor. The government considers almost everything that goes into a person's bank account or wallet to be income, whether taxable or not. If it remains in the wallet or bank account at the end of the month, it's an asset in the following month.

The federal income entitlement program is *Social Security OASDI* – Old Age (retirement), Survivor (and dependent), and Disability Income (SSDI). Social Security retirement or disability is an entitlement because the person receiving such payments paid Social Security taxes. These benefits were promised when the taxes were enacted and collected. Or, one is entitled to a dependent or survivor check after one's parent or spouse retires, becomes disabled, or dies—but only if that parent or spouse paid Social Security taxes. There are other eligibility criteria, which you can find on the Social Security Administration's website (www.ssa.gov).

The federal healthcare entitlement program for those with a disability is Medicare. One is entitled to Medicare because, if less than 65 old, one has received a Social Security disability check for 24 consecutive months (which means someone—either the person with disabilities herself or a parent—paid Social Security taxes).

The federal need-based income program is *Supplemental Security Income* (SSI). There is not an income limit per se to receive SSI, but receiving other types of income will reduce the SSI check either by 50 percent (earned income such as wages from a job) or by 100 percent (unearned income such as monetary gifts or interest from a bank account). In 2011, the maximum SSI payment was $674 per month.

The federal need-based healthcare program is *Medicaid,* which also covers assisted living or skilled nursing for the elderly or disabled. Medicaid has an income limit to qualify—$2,094 per month (2012) in most states for an individual. Eighty-six percent of Medicaid expenditures support children, the disabled, and the frail elderly—people who need help through no fault of their own.

Both SSI and Medicaid have a limit on the financial assets one may have and yet be eligible for benefits. It is $2,000, a number that is not indexed to inflation. It is this number that drives much of what is done in special needs financial planning.

It is important to be aware of the *"deeming rule."* Earlier, when explaining guardianship, I mentioned that a minor child becomes an adult at his or her eighteenth birthday. Parents have a legal obligation to support their minor child. Thus, Social Security and Medicaid authorities "deem" the parents' income and assets to also be the income and assets of the child. Consequently, children aged birth through age 17 of living, pre-retirement, nondisabled parents will not be eligible for SSI, Medicaid, or state services unless the entire family lives in poverty. But at age 18, only the child's income and assets can be deemed to them. Most children with DS-ASD will become eligible for SSI, Medicaid, and state services upon their eighteenth birthday.

Social Security and SSI and Medicare and Medicaid are complicated programs. You should be aware of the benefits and eligibility criteria. The Social Security Administration and the Center for Medicare and Medicaid Services have excellent websites and good publications explaining how things work.

State Government Programs

Disability services are also delivered at the state level. Typically these are what are called HCBS Programs—Home and Community Based Services Programs. A variety of services are provided by the states (sometimes only theoretically)—a residence, job assistance, care and supervision, case management, transportation, community day programs, and respite care. A key thing to know is that most states use Medicaid's eligibility requirement for state service eligibility. The most important eligibility requirement is the $2,000 asset limit.

The cost of state comprehensive services for an individual with a moderate or more severe developmental disability typically runs from $60,000-$120,000 per year. Only the most affluent of families can afford to pay this amount to support their child with special needs—especially one with moderate, severe, or profound needs—without government assistance. Consequently, an essential element of financial and legal planning for most families will be assuring that the child maintains government benefit eligibility as an adult. The $2,000 asset limit dominates special needs planning.

Resource Plan - Private Pay

Most parents, to the extent they can afford it, will want to do more for their child than to leave them to the mercy—or neglect—of the state. Most families have to dip into "private pay" resources for one of three reasons. The first reason is because the child can't get services because of inadequate state funding—the infamous problem of state "wait lists," which in my state (Colorado) has become a "die list." A second reason is to supplement state services when capped. For example, you may be told your child can only get "300 units" (whatever that means) of speech therapy. When you exhaust your 300 units, the rest is out of your wallet. The third reason is to provide a service or product that the state will not pay for; for example, a handicap-modified automobile.

Typically, "private pay" resources fall in these basic areas:

- Disability-related expenses that the state chooses not to cover or won't pay for because of inadequate funding or caps on benefits
- Private residential options, including an apartment, condominium, or home
- Opening doors to better employment opportunities through secondary education, vocational training, or employment placement and assistance
- Personal care and support, skilled or unskilled, ranging from paid companions to skilled care managers. Expenses for professional services can be substantial if the child outlives his or her parents.

For children capable of semi-independent living and employment, the resources to enable such independence become important elements of the resource plan. They often become dominant elements of expense, but for reasons of space we cannot go further here. Enabling employment and semi-independent living presents significant challenges.

Financial Plan

Special needs financial planning addresses how much support the child will need and how that support can be provided while maintaining eligibility for government need-based services. Because the desired quality of life must be affordable, there are typically two financial plans—a plan for the family and a plan for the child with special needs.

The child's financial plan typically addresses:

- An estimate of the amount needed for lifelong financial support
- Structuring financial arrangements to meet income and asset eligibility limits for "need-based" government assistance; this often includes establishing a special needs trust and using proper title for gifts, assets, bequests, and insurance death or disability benefits to transfer money or assets to the trust
- Funding a special needs trust—how much, when, and with what
- Tracing the flow of estate distributions at the death of either or both parents to assure the special needs child is taken care of and doesn't directly receive an unforeseen bequest or death benefit that would cause her to lose her government assistance

The family's financial plan addresses:

- How much support can be provided in fairness to all of the children
- How to assure the parents' life goals are also met, such as their retirement
- Efficient wealth accumulation to improve the quality of life for all family members, including that of the special needs child
- Protecting the family and the special needs child by assuring that the income and care providers have adequate health, life, disability, and long-term care insurance

Legal (or Estate) Plan

Legal planning involves the preparation and execution of the legal documents that will assure the parents' wishes are carried out when they die or become disabled. Two important documents are personal wills and a special needs trust agreement.

Choosing a Lawyer: There are two types of attorneys qualified for special needs planning: an elder law attorney or a trusts and estates (T&E) attorney. I recommend elder law attorneys because they are required to have expertise in the laws and regulations for Social Security, Medicare, Medicaid, and state disability services. (The frail elderly are people with special needs.) An elder law attorney will almost always know how to draft a legally-conforming special needs trust. Most trusts and estates attorneys are also expert in this area, but some are not. If you are contemplating working with a trust and estates attorney, inquire as to his or her experience with drafting special needs trusts and special needs estate plans.

Wills: Both parents should have wills. The primary purpose of a will is to assure that your assets pass to whom you wish upon your death unless you have made a legally acceptable alternative arrangement. However, there is a crucial provision when there is a special needs child. It is the designation of a *successor guardian,* should both parents die together, or one predeceases and the surviving parent forgets to update their will naming the deceased parent. The state presumes, absent someone establishing otherwise, that the natural parents of a minor child (up to age 18) are the appropriate guardians. So who will the state appoint as guardians of a special needs child (if ap-

propriate) when the natural parents die? The courts generally accept the wishes of the parents unless someone presents a convincing reason not to. How does the court know what the parents' wishes are? The preferred way is to designate your choice of a successor guardian in a properly executed will. Your primary successor guardian will likely be your spouse, unless you are single. It is also important to designate a secondary successor guardian, in the event your spouse dies before you or at the same time. When the will is probated, the guardianship order will be issued as an outcome of the probate process.

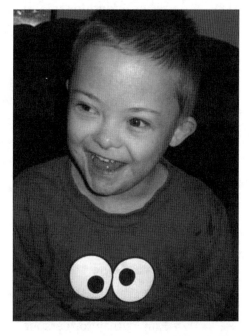

Trusts: An estate plan for a family with a special needs child will almost always include establishing a special needs trust if the family plans on need-based government assistance—SSI, Medicaid, and state disability services. A properly drafted, legally-conforming special needs trust allows a family—parents, grandparents, siblings, and others—to set aside money to support a loved one that will not be counted in the $2,000 asset limit.

The trust pays for additional or supplemental benefits not provided by the government. (A special needs trust is also called a supplemental needs trust.) Payments made by the trust are usually made directly to providers of goods and services and not to the beneficiary so that such payments are *not* counted as the child's income, and therefore do not reduce or eliminate SSI or eliminate Medicaid eligibility.

In order for the government to accept that the assets in the trust are not assets of the individual with disabilities, the individual cannot have any right to force a payment, or have any control over the assets, or have any legal right to modify or terminate the trust. If the person with disabilities can't get at the assets, then the government can't consider them to belong to the person. Thus the trustee of a special needs trust must have absolute discretion to make distributions for the individual's benefit. He or she (or it, in the case of a bank or trust company) cannot have any legal obligation to make payments but can have guidance as to when payments are appropriate. To satisfy this requirement of Social Security, Medicaid, and state laws, the trust must be drafted with legally bullet-proof language. You should absolutely have the trust drafted by a competent attorney—an elder law or a trust and estates attorney.

Communicating Your Plan to Others

Once you have your special needs plan, you will need to create a Letter of Intent (LOI). A letter of intent documents the life, resource, financial, and legal plans you have made. It describes what you want and what you have arranged; and the needs, capabilities, and wishes of the child. It is not a legally binding document, but I have found that those who will be involved with your child's care, support, or protection are usually grateful for such guidance and will follow it. The key people who should have copies of your letter of intent are the personal representative for your estate, successor guardians, and trustees and the primary care manager.

The content includes both the current arrangements that will continue and the arrangements that will have to be made after your death. Topics your LOI should address include, as appropriate:

- Personal information about the child or adult with disabilities
- Key people in the child's life
- Medical needs
- Social life
- Spiritual life
- Residential environment
- Education
- Employment or personal business
- Social Security benefits
- Medicaid benefits
- State disability or vocational services
- Estate plans and legal documents
- Financial arrangements, including investment accounts and insurance
- Final arrangements for when the child dies

What does an LOI look like? It is three things: a cover letter, backup files, and a personal narrative. The cover letter summarizes your special needs plan, by element or topic, noting how to reach key people and where to find backup documents or files. The backup files are folders in a filing cabinet. To the extent possible, I suggest you keep everything in one place. The personal narrative is a description of your child's needs and capabilities, her wishes for herself, and how you care for her. One of the best personal narratives I have seen was a letter detailing a week in the life of a severely challenged child prepared by her mother. It described the child as a person, including biographical and personal sketches. It described the child's daily schedule and activities. It described all of the tasks that the mother and her husband performed for the child's care and support. The personal narrative was a picture of the life of that family in a typical week.

The Twelve Essential Steps in Special Needs Planning

In closing, there are twelve things you should remember as you plan for your child's future, twelve steps. If you take care of these twelve things, you likely have an acceptable comprehensive special needs plan:

1. Start with a life plan.
2. Get serious about planning when your child is in middle school. Earlier is much better.
3. Understand the eligibility requirements for SSI, Medicaid, and state disability services.
4. Sign up for state services as soon as permitted so your child can take her place on the state "wait lists."
5. Consider the appointment of successor guardians, care managers, and fiduciaries (trustees, trust protector, and those holding a power-of-attorney) and how they will work together.
6. Engage an attorney and a financial advisor with current knowledge of Social Security, Medicare, and laws and regulations for Medicaid and state disability services.
7. Execute wills; set up a special needs trust if you intend to use government assistance.
8. Use proper titles and designations for gifts, bequests, and death benefits to assure asset transfers are made to the special needs trust and not directly to the child.
9. Have a strategy to open doors to employment.
10. Consider the full range of residential options—public and private—including home ownership.
11. Document your life plan, your wishes, your child's wishes, and your arrangements in a letter of intent.
12. Review your plan and letter of intent at least annually, update them as needed, and keep them current.

My best wishes for you and your loved one with DS-ASD.

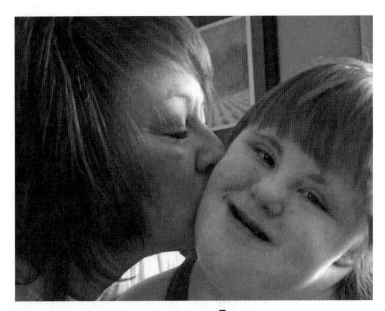

15

Finding Support and Encouragement for the Journey
Advice from a Seasoned Parent

Robin Zaborek

The Analogy of the Jump Ropes

When I was a little girl, throngs of neighborhood kids would congregate in the cul-de-sac and play outside all day until the streetlights came on. We played all sorts of games, making many of them up as we went along. We would ride bikes, play "kick the can," catch salamanders under drainage bridges, make up cheers and perform them, and, of course, we would jump rope.

At first we would line up with our own ropes and have contests to see who could go the longest without tripping, counting out loud at the top of our lungs, and then when someone did trip we would yell, "OUT!" and that person would go to the back of the line. Then we graduated to longer ropes where two friends would hold the ends and we would jump in the middle. Our friends would always play tricks, like going too fast, wiggling the rope on the ground like a snake, or lowering the rope quickly and unexpectedly. We learned so much playing games like these. At first there was lots of tripping and losing. Then we all got really good at it.

One day, someone introduced a second jump rope to the mix. That's when the friends at either end held two ropes and twirled them at different intervals. Now *that* was a challenge. As with every other jump-rope game we played, we tripped and made a lot of mistakes in the beginning. We wished that our friend had never brought the second rope. We felt uncomfortable and embarrassed at our incompetence, and we were called "out" a million times before we got the hang of it.

But we did get the hang of it, and eventually we were all pretty fancy jumpers. We would hop on one leg, turn around mid-jump, and sing elaborate jumping chants. We learned through trial and error how to manage the double ropes coming at our feet. After a while we simply got into a rhythm, and our confidence blossomed. We became experts.

When we have a baby born with Down syndrome, it's like someone handing us a rope and saying, "Here, become an expert at this. This is your rope now. Someday it will be fun." But we didn't ask for that rope. We look at others who can use the rope well, and we think, "That will never be me." We grieve, we examine the rope (it's a beautiful rope), we look on the Internet at every jump-rope website we can find, and, with a bit of apprehension, we give it a try. At first we trip and fall a bit, but eventually we start to get the hang of it. We meet people who are already really good at this game, and we seek their advice. In time, we are finding our rhythm. We trip less and less. It not only becomes easier; we start to look like we actually know what we're doing.

Then one day, that second jump rope is introduced. The second jump rope is autism. Perhaps we've seen that other rope hanging around. We've noticed it. We've poked at it. We've wondered why it's there and we hoped that it would just go away. It doesn't help much that there are people who say that they can't even see the second rope. Maybe we're imagining it. But why would we imagine a rope that we don't even want?

We ask question after question until finally someone confirms our fears. Suddenly, this second rope has been officially added to our game: it's heavy and cumbersome, a burden we didn't desire, but it was placed into our hands nonetheless. We have no choice in the matter now; we must gather our courage and learn how to jump over two ropes. The pace gets faster and faster. At first we feel clumsy, but we stay with it. We remind ourselves that it's just a matter of finding the right rhythm, and we've done it before.

In time we are rockin' the newer, more complicated rhythm, and we are regaining our confidence. Now all we need to do is to find others who also jump double ropes. We observe them and pose questions. We listen and learn how to avoid the pitfalls. It feels nice just knowing that someone else knows what it's like to play this game. Maybe someday we will be able to help people who are new to this game and teach them all the tricks to becoming experts—like we are now. And we want them to learn how to love jumping rope, because even though it's really hard at times, the game truly brings a joy that we never would have known if these ropes had never been given to us.

Where to Find Support

There are many ways in which you may find support and comfort. The first thing to understand is that you are not alone. It may feel tremendously lonely at times; however, there are others in this world jumping double ropes, and they are not strangers to the joys and challenges of living with DS-ASD. You do not have to "go it alone." Allow yourself to be encouraged, and remember that parents are each other's best resources.

Use Technology to Find Support

No matter where you live, you can find others who understand and care about your journey. In this day and age, social media can connect even those living in the most remote areas to other people who are living with DS-ASD. You can find online support groups (such as ds-autism@yahoogroups.com), post questions on Facebook and websites (such as the Down Syndrome-Autism Connection's Facebook page and website at http://ds-asd-connection.org), and read blogs by other parents who are living with DS-ASD. You might be pleasantly surprised if you take the initiative and reach out for help. You can find others in distant cities who know how to jump two ropes and make an emotional connection with them.

Be Open to Using Respite Care

As parents raising children and adults with DS-ASD, it is imperative that we get a break now and then. We must find opportunities to get some time away from all the jumping and use some different muscles for a while. A brief reprieve from our daily care giving duties is called respite. Respite can be anything from going grocery shopping alone (no meltdowns) to enjoy-ing dinner and a movie with a spouse or friend, or even getting away for the weekend. Respite is basically doing anything that brings you joy and gives you a break from thinking about Down syndrome and autism for a little while.

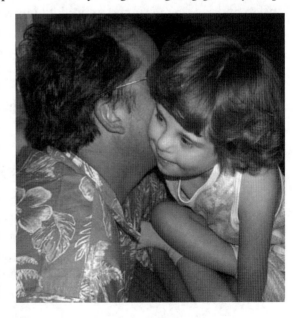

There is no shame in taking a break to recharge your batteries. In fact, finding respite care is a responsible way to strengthen your family, your other relationships, and your ability to be a better parent for the long haul. And this may surprise you, but your child might also enjoy a break from you from time to time. If you don't have anyone in your life who can stay with your child, you may be able to find respite programs in your community. Some disability organizations (such as local branches of the Arc or Easter Seals) offer respite opportunities with professional care-givers, and they may even provide funding as an added incentive. Another idea may be to find another parent in your area who needs respite and to create a respite "co-op" by taking care of each other's child. This way, you can arrange to take each other's ropes for a short time so you can both get a break.

Ask for Help from Your Local Support Groups

If your area has a local Down syndrome support group and/or Autism Society chapter, ask if they have a specialized outreach for families dealing with dual diagno-ses, or if they would be willing to start one, perhaps collaboratively. Or find a group elsewhere, such as the Down Syndrome-Autism Connection™ (http://ds-asd-connec-tion.org), and ask how they may provide some long-distance support.

Seek Opportunities for Support through Your Faith Community

While many people find solace in their faith, some families with children/adults with DS-ASD find it difficult to attend their place of worship because of their child's behaviors and the noises he makes, so they forego the experience completely. This can make families feel even more isolated and leave them without the spiritual support they feel they need. Some people have found, however, that simply by asking, some-one is willing to help them find ways to attend service. Perhaps that means asking a member to provide volunteer respite care in your home, or possibly to watch your child in another room in the building so you can be close by if you are needed. Others are able to find services designed for individuals with developmental disabilities and their families. If there is no such opportunity where you live, maybe there is someone who would be willing to develop one—if they only knew there was a need.

Remember, there are a lot of people out there who have no idea what it is like to jump double ropes. They don't even know how to jump one rope. Sometimes a little education goes a long way, and after people gain a better understanding, they may be more willing to help.

Find an Advocate Who Knows Your Child

Find a professional, or professionals, who will advocate for you. It's always com-forting to know that there is someone in your corner, whether a pediatrician, teacher, classroom aide, therapist, etc. It is best to maintain a level of professional respect, how-ever, so please do not monopolize your advocates' time and resources. In other words, you may feel very close and friendly over time, but wait for their cues. If they haven't asked you to call them by their first name, then don't. Maintain appropriate boundaries.

Remain positive and easy to work with. Parents who become militant or too demanding risk alienating the very people they will need to depend on in the future. Yes, be a strong advocate for your child *always*, but keep in mind that you will benefit greatly from developing influential allies who care about your DS-ASD journey.

Find a Confidant

A confidant can be your spouse, a close friend, a family member, a member of the clergy—anyone who will listen to you vent your feelings without bringing judgment against you or your child. Your confidant will not criticize you if you're tripping on your ropes, and he or she won't call you a "saint" when you are in your perfect rhythm. Your confidant must be your safe place for expressing your sadness during tough times as well as the person who rejoices with you when your child succeeds.

Surround Yourself with Positive People

Surround yourself with people who are helpful and upbeat about your child with DS-ASD. Conversely, restrict contact with those who are negative about your child or who pity you. The people you choose to spend time with should be cheering you on and applauding your jump-rope abilities. You do not need someone breathing down your neck who is pessimistic about your jump-rope skills or about your child's DS-ASD forcing you to play this game.

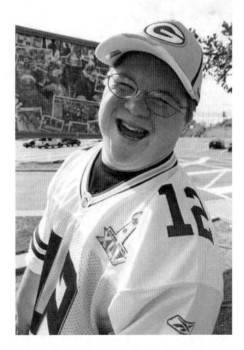

Your child is precious and beautiful, and his disabilities are only a part of who he is. Please focus on what your child can do, not on what he can't do. And remember, what he can't do yet, he may someday master. No one has a crystal ball, so don't buy into the "nevers." My daughter, Janet Kay, could have easily been considered extremely "low functioning," yet she still had the ability to completely astonish us in new and unexpected ways. She disproved a lot of pessimists with her determination! And if I had bought into the "nevers," I wouldn't have watched for the intelligence hiding behind her autism. Our family had high expectations for her, and Janet Kay achieved far more than anyone had ever predicted for her life.

Be Patient with Yourself

It may seem "easier said than done" to find that rhythmic groove that brings predictability and comfort to our lives as parents raising kids with DS-ASD, and I don't blame you if you are a bit skeptical. Admittedly, it takes a lot of hard work and selflessness, and the tiniest thing can throw us off our rhythm. Be aware of your own grief and how it may appear unexpectedly, out of nowhere. Be aware that there will be tough days as well as days that bring you genuine joy. If you're having a hard day, seek opportunities for support and respite. Remind yourself that no parent is perfect, and pat yourself on the back for the amazing job that you are doing in raising your child.

Yes, the challenges that DS-ASD brings to our lives can seem insurmountable at times. However, what I've learned from my many years of working with parents of children with developmental disabilities is that we possess a resilience, strength, creativity, and determination second to none. And, we love our children with a ferocity that simultaneously breaks our hearts and fills us with a pride we cannot possibly describe. Be encouraged, my friends . . . we are all on this journey together.

About the Contributors

Kimberly Bonello is a mother of three children; her youngest child is a young adult with DS-ASD. Kim was the founder and facilitator for Parent Advocates Lending Support (P.A.L.S.) Support Group. Kim is involved in the Down Syndrome-Autism Connection™ in Colorado, providing support to other parents who are newer to the DS-ASD diagnosis.

Brian Chicoine, MD, is the Medical Director of the Adult Down Syndrome Center of Lutheran General Hospital and on the faculty of Family Practice at Lutheran General Hospital of Advocate Health Care in Park Ridge, Illinois. Dr. Chicoine is cofounder of the Adult Down Syndrome Center. This Center has served and documented the health and psychosocial needs of over 4500 adults with Down syndrome since its inception in 1992. Dr. Chicoine graduated from Loyola University Stritch School of Medicine and completed his Family Practice residency at Lutheran General Hospital. He has provided medical care for adults with developmental disabilities for more than 16 years. He presents regularly at national and international conferences, has published numerous articles, and has coauthored two books, *Mental Wellness in Adults with Down Syndrome* and *The Guide to Good Health for Teens and Adults with Down Syndrome* (Woodbine House).

Ellen Roy Elias, MD, FAAP, FACMG, is the Director of The Special Care Clinic at Children's Hospital Colorado, where she provides both primary and consultative care to children with developmental disabilities and a variety of complex special health care needs. She is Board Certified in Pediatrics, Clinical Genetics, and Neurodevelopmental Disabilities. In addition to patient care, she is also actively involved in clinical research. She studies a rare cause of autism called Smith-Lemli-Opitz Syndrome (SLOS) and was one of the discoverers of the cause of this genetic disorder. She is interested in the underlying genetic etiologies of autism, and is part of a multi-institutional study funded by the CDC called CADDRE, which is studying the physical features of children with autism. She is also using innovative genetic technology to study the genetic etiologies of autism in patients with Down syndrome.

Dr. Elias enjoys teaching fellows, pediatric residents, and medical students about Down syndrome. She is also mentoring a medical student who is studying how doctors learn to care for patients with Down syndrome. She enjoys writing and has published many articles and chapters in textbooks. She was an editor of the most recent edition of the textbook *Developmental-Behavioral Pediatrics,* 4th Edition (Elsevier, 2008).

Deborah J. Fidler, PhD, is Associate Professor of Human Development and Family Studies, Colorado State University. She also holds a clinical faculty position in the Department of Pediatrics at the University of Colorado Health Sciences Center. She earned a BS in Psychology from Cornell University and an MS and PhD in Psychological Studies in Education from the University of California, Los Angeles. Her research focuses on development in children with genetic disorders, with a focus on emerging behavioral phenotypes, family outcomes, and early intervention strategies.

Margaret Froehlke, RN, BSN, is the mother of four children, one of whom has both Down syndrome and autism spectrum disorder (DS-ASD). Margaret and her family moved to Denver from Michigan in 2008. Froehlke worked as Executive Director of the Denver Adult Down Syndrome Clinic, and is now on staff with Adam's Camp. Additional work experiences include the Autism Society of Michigan, pediatric hospital nursing, corporate, and nonprofit positions with a focus on health and human services, and community-based work focused on inclusion. Margaret is also the author of *Mass, A Guide for Visual Learners,* a book designed to assist persons with ASD in attending the Catholic Mass. Margaret received her Bachelor of Science in Nursing (BSN) from Wayne State University and is a Registered Licensed Nurse in Colorado.

Robert Froehlke, MD, graduated from the University of Notre Dame (magna cum laude), and received his M.D. from St. Louis University. He completed a residency in pediatrics at Northwestern University/Children's Memorial Hospital, and a fellowship in epidemiology and public health at the Centers for Disease Control. He has served in a number of different and varied professional positions, including: an assistant to the U.S. Surgeon General, assistant professor of pediatrics at Michigan State University School of Medicine, Commander in the Medical Corps of the United States Naval Reserve, and Director of Sparrow Hospital inpatient pediatric service in Lansing, Michigan. He is a fellow in the American Academy of Pediatrics, and member of the Down Syndrome Medical Interest Group (DSMIG). He has received several awards, authored/co-authored many publications, and given numerous presentations.

Dr. Froehlke is currently in private pediatric practice in Littleton, CO, where he specializes in general pediatrics, as well as the care of children with Down Syndrome, autism, and other disabilities. He is married to Margaret Froehlke and has four children, including a son, Brennan, who has Down syndrome and autism spectrum disorder.

Sarah Hartway, RN, MS, holds the following positions: Vice-President, Down Syndrome Pregnancy, Inc.; Executive Board member of the Down Syndrome-Autism Connection; formerly Director of Professional Partnerships at Mile High Down Syndrome Association; Developer of the Mile High Down Syndrome Association's Health Care Partnership, one of the first and largest Down syndrome healthcare outreach programs in the country; Clinical Instructor, University of Colorado at Denver, College of Nursing; Down Syndrome Affiliates in Action, Informed Decision Making Task Force member. Ms. Hartway is also a parent of three, including a teenage son with Down syndrome. In addition, Sarah has authored and/or co-authored several publications, including: "Family Teaching Toolbox – Down Syndrome," *Advances in Neonatal Care* (Feb. 2009); "A Parent's Guide to the Genetics of Down Syndrome," *Advances in Neonatal Care* (Feb. 2009); "Ancient History or Current Practice?", *The Colorado Pediatrician* (2003).

Susan Hepburn, PhD, Clinical Psychology (Vanderbilt University), is an Associate Professor of Psychiatry and Pediatrics at the University of Colorado School of Medicine. She is the Director of Research at JFK Partners, which is the University Center for Excellence in Developmental Disabilities for the Front Range region. Dr. Hepburn's research focuses on the development of children with different developmental disabilities, with a particular interest in co-occurring conditions. Dr. Hepburn also teaches courses in assessment, ethics, and research methods through the Leadership and Education in Neurodevelopmental Disorders program at the University of Colorado. She works directly with families and schools across the state.

Fran Hickey, MD, was recently appointed the medical director of the Anna and John J. Sie Center for Down Syndrome at The Colorado Children's Hospital. A developmental pediatrician by training, Dr. Hickey was a Boston native, educated at Harvard University and the University of Cincinnati College of Medicine. Trained at Cincinnati Children's in pediatrics and Boston Children's in developmental behavioral pediatrics, Dr. Hickey has spent over 20 years as a developmental pediatrician in private practice and an adjunct Assistant Professor of Pediatrics at the University of Cincinnati College of Medicine. For the past ten years, he conducted clinical evaluations and research involving individuals with Down syndrome at the Cincinnati Children's Hospital Medical Center. In addition, Dr. Hickey has published numerous articles on Down syndrome and autism. Dr. Hickey and his wife also have personal experience on the subject, being the parents of a son, James, with DS-ASD.

Terry Katz, PhD, is a Senior Instructor and licensed psychologist in the Department of Pediatrics at the University of Colorado School of Medicine. Dr. Katz provides assessment and treatment for children and families through her work at the Autism and Developmental Disabilities Clinic at JFK Partners and at the Child Development Unit at the Children's Hospital. She has worked with children with developmental disabilities since 1986. She has an interest in diagnostic evaluation tools and provides training and supervision in assessment measures. Dr. Katz is involved in the Autism Treatment Network (ATN), a network of collaborative clinical teams that provides ongoing care to children and families at sites across the United States and Canada. Dr. Katz will assist in the implementation of a study that will investigate the effectiveness of parent-based sleep education programs. She co-leads a sleep clinic for children with autism at the Child Development Unit and works as a sleep psychologist in the Pulmonary Clinic at the Children's Hospital.

Elina R. Manghi, PsyD, LMFT (1952-2012), was a family therapist and child psychologist who helped create a support group in Chicago for Spanish-speaking families with autistic children in 2003 called Groupo SALTO. She was formerly a clinical professor in the department of disability and human development at the University of Illinois at Chicago, and co-director of The Autism Program. The author of many publications based on her research and clinical work in the United States and internationally, particularly on the topic of autism, Elina was a strong supporter and dear friend of the Down Syndrome-Autism Connection.

Dennis McGuire, PhD, is the Director of Psychosocial Services for the Adult Down Syndrome Center of Lutheran General Hospital, in suburban Chicago. Dr. McGuire helped to establish the Adult Down Syndrome Center, which has served the health and psychosocial needs of over 4,500 adults with Down syndrome since its inception in 1992. Dr. McGuire received his master's degree from the University of Chicago and his doctorate from the University of Illinois at Chicago. His work experience includes over 30 years in mental health and developmental disabilities. He presents regularly at national and international conferences, has published numerous articles, and has coauthored two books, *Mental Wellness of Adults with Down Syndrome* and *The Guide to Good Health for Teens and Adults with Down Syndrome* (Woodbine House).

Patti McVay has a B.S. in Psychology with a focus on students with severe disabilities and a Master of Science in Education, Special Education. Patti has taught high school and served as a principal at both the elementary and postsecondary levels during her career. In each of these positions, Patti provided leadership and direction to create inclusive school communities for all students, including those with intellectual, physical, and other disabilities. Patti has extensive experience working with children with Down syndrome and has provided training in Oregon, California, Kansas, Florida, Massachusetts, Utah, and New York. Patti has authored several articles, training materials, and books, including *Ideas, Samples & Designs: Best Practices for Inclusive Education* (2003) and *Ideas, Samples & Designs: Helping All Students Learn Successfully in General Education* (2001). She currently is a special education director in Santa Rosa, CA.

Susan Merrill, MD, graduated with honors from the University of Colorado School of Medicine in 1980. She has been a pediatrician for Kaiser Permanente for 30 years, and served as department chief for 5 years. Throughout her career as a pediatrician, Dr. Merrill has mentored many medical students and pediatric residents, and is a clinical professor of pediatrics for the University of Colorado Health Sciences Center. Her practice includes a number of patients with complex medical issues, each requiring a true teamwork approach with the family.

Laura Pickler, MD, MPH, is Assistant Professor of Family Medicine, Pediatric Genetics, and Otolaryngology at the University of Colorado School of Medicine, Children's Hospital Colorado/University of Colorado Hospital, and Director of Pediatric Oral Feeding Clinic, Special Care Clinic, Compass Clinic. Dr. Laura Pickler is a family physician with an active primary care practice serving children, youth, and young adults with special health care needs. She also has completed two medical fellowships in Child Development and Clinical Genetics and Metabolism and additionally provides consultative care in these fields. Prior to attending medical school, she completed a Master's Degree in Public Health nutrition with the goal of becoming a dietitian. Combined, this training has poised her to take a lead role in implementing medical homes for children and adults who are underserved in the community. She understands first-hand the challenges of providing comprehensive, coordinated care that creatively works with diverse family dynamics.

In addition to her clinical expertise, Dr. Pickler serves as the physician consultant for her state public health department program for children with special needs. She also has ongoing academic research interests. She is a frequently requested national speaker on medical homes and transition needs of youth with special health care needs. In her spare time, she teaches medical students and residents at the University of Colorado School of Medicine.

Ann Reynolds, MD, received a BS in biology at Emory University, an MD at Medical College of Georgia, and completed a Residency in Pediatrics at Children's National Medical Center/George Washington University, and a Fellowship in Neurodevelopmental Disabilities at Texas Children's Hospital/Baylor College of Medicine. Dr. Reynolds, Assistant Professor in Pediatrics at the University of Colorado at Denver and Health Sciences Center, is a developmental pediatrician for JFK Partners at the Child Development.

Cordelia Robinson, PhD, RN, BS, has been director of JFK Partners, an interdepartmental program of Pediatrics and Psychiatry at the Colorado University School of

Medicine, since 1993. In this role she is responsible for providing leadership and direction to an interdisciplinary professional staff of over forty faculty members. Dr. Robinson has professional preparation in Nursing (BS) and Special Education (MA) from D'Youville College in Buffalo, NY, and in Developmental Psychology, with a research specialty in Intellectual Disabilities (PhD) from Peabody College of Vanderbilt University. She is currently Professor of Pediatrics, Psychiatry and Preventative Medicine.

Dr. Robinson has worked in the field of early intervention for children with developmental disabilities as a clinician, researcher, and educator of personnel from multiple disciplines since 1973. She has been the principal investigator on over 30 federally funded demonstration, training, or research projects in the field of Developmental Disabilities and Intellectual Disabilities. Since 2001, her work has been focused on autism spectrum disorders. She is Co-Principal Investigator on the CDCP-funded Colorado CADDRE and Surveillance projects and Co-Principal Investigator on the Colorado site of the Autism Treatment Network. Her community work in Colorado includes service on the Developmental Disabilities Council and the Colorado Autism Commission.

Kirsti Seibel, DMD, started her career in dentistry as Dr. Tesini's patient. While in high school she worked as Dr. Tesini's dental assistant and she continued in the dental field while completing her bachelor's degree at the University of Massachusetts at Amherst. She earned her DMD degree from Tufts University School of Dental Medicine in Boston. While earning her DMD degree, Dr. Seibel was an officer in the Smile Squad, an extracurricular children's dental health education outreach program. After working some years as a general dentist, Dr. Seibel returned to Tufts to specialize in her first love, pediatric dentistry. Her training included treating children, young adults, and special needs patients at New England Medical Center, the Cotting School, and Brookline Dept. of Health Dental Clinic. Dr. Seibel is a Diplomate of the American Board of Pediatric Dentistry. Currently, Dr. Seibel is working with the Massachusetts Dental Society Leadership Institution to educate caregivers of persons with special needs about dental care. She is also a Gold Award Scout and life member of the Girl Scouts of America, as well as a proud mother of two children.

David A. Tesini, DMD, MS, FDS, RCSEd, is a pediatric dentist and Associate Clinical Professor at Tufts University, School of Dental Medicine. He has served as Associate-Chief-Dentist at Tufts Dental Facilities for Patients with Special Needs. His administrative, clinical, and teaching responsibilities have included development and direction of three clinics for patients with disabilities; supervising preventive and research activities of students; and national and international lecturing on prevention, early orthodontic treatment, dental care for patients with special needs, and management of children's behavior in pediatric dentistry. He has published over 20 articles in refereed scientific journals, texts, monographs, and manuals.

Dr. Tesini has served in various capacities for statewide and national organizations including appointment as the Massachusetts Dental Society's Chairman of Council on Dental Health, past president of the American Academy of Dentistry for Persons with Disabilities, Treasurer of the Federation of Special Care Organizations in Dentistry, and the American Dental Association's representative to the Joint Commission of Health Care Organizations. In his capacity as chairman of the MDS Council on Dental Health, he developed the statewide access program ("Dentistry for All") for indigent families in Massachusetts. He is the founder and past president of Project Stretch: Dentistry Reaching Out to Children, a nonprofit foundation providing free dental care to children around the world. Over 20,000 children have received preventive and sustaining dental care from over 200 Project Stretch volunteers since 1986.

Sam Towers, M.Ed., owner of Towers Behavior Services, LLC, is a behavior analyst who has spent 21 years providing support to individuals with disabilities who use problem behavior. In addition, he has served as a special educator and has trained special education teachers at the University of Kentucky. Sam has a Master's Degree in special education from the University of Northern Colorado and has completed three years of post-master's training at the University of Kentucky. Sam welcomes invitations to serve in other nations, especially developing nations.

Hal Wright, CFP®, has been married thirty-nine years and has three adult children, one born with Down syndrome. He received a Bachelor of Science degree from Tulane University, School of Engineering, and an MBA from Loyola University of the South. He is an LPL Financial Planner and Investment Advisor Representative and is affiliated with Colorado Financial Partners, LLC. He is a Certified Financial Planner™ and a recognized expert in special needs planning. He published a book in 2009: *Special Needs Planning for a Person with a Disability: Life, Resource, Financial & Legal*. He is frequently invited to speak, locally and nationally, to nonprofit organizations, schools, churches, parent groups, and professional societies on this subject.

Robin Zaborek is a proud mother of four children, including an adult son with Down syndrome and a teenage daughter with Down syndrome and autism (DS-ASD), Janet Kay, who passed away during the final stages of writing this book. Robin has a Bachelor of Arts degree from Beloit College, is a CDA (Child Development Associate), is a CNA (Certified Nurse's Assistant) for her daughter, and is a long-time advocate for people with developmental disabilities. Robin is a cofounder of the Down Syndrome-Autism Connection™, whose mission is to provide support and education to families and professionals impacted by DS-ASD. Her passion is helping families and providers receive the support and education they need—with the ultimate goal being that children and adults living with DS-ASD and other developmental disabilities will receive the understanding, education, medical care, and opportunities they so greatly deserve.

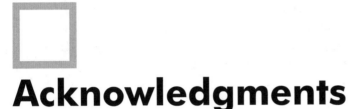

Acknowledgments

Margaret Froehlke, BSN, RN:

Throughout Brennan's life, our family's journey has been blessed and touched by many, beginning with our large extended family. My thanks and appreciation for the time taken and love offered to make the special connections with Brennan that have given him such joy and a fuller life.

Our walk with Brennan has been supported by an incredible team of educators since he was six weeks of age. Thank you all for your time, talents, patience, love, and support.

Thank you to all Brennan's school friends from Haslett, Michigan to Centennial, Colorado. Your kindness, sense of humor, respect, and interest in Brennan means the world to him and us.

Finally, to my family, Liz, Buddy, Sarah, and especially my husband, Bob—who gives me inspiration every day through his humble example—thank you for the love, support, and encouragement you gave to help make this dream project a reality.

Robin Sattel Zaborek:

My heartfelt appreciation goes out to all the amazing people who have contributed their expertise to this book. I am humbled and honored that you took part, and I am grateful beyond words.

Thank you to Dr. Susan Merrill, for being a constant source of level-headed support in our lives—through the good, the bad, and the ugly—for over twenty-six years. Thank you for your extraordinary compassion after Tommy was born with Down syndrome, and for your support when I told you years later that we wanted to adopt an unborn baby girl with Down syndrome. Thank you for being her pediatrician when she arrived on the scene with more medical issues than we had bargained for, and later after she was diagnosed with a whopping case of autism. You are our hero.

Thank you to my dear family, friends, and mentors who have held me up throughout my DS-ASD journey. There are too many of you to name, but you know who you are! I hope I can lean on you for many years to come.

Of course, I send my biggest thanks to my husband, Robert, and to our family, Joey, Rebekah, Asher, Tommy, Caroline, and Janet Kay, for being my soul mates on this rollercoaster ride. Our intense love for each other—and your ability to make me laugh every single day—have made my life worth living.

Index